FAREWELL JET LAG

Cures from a Flight Attendant

T0333231

Christopher
Babayode

Farewell Jet Lag

First published in 2016 by

Panoma Press Ltd
48 St Vincent Drive, St Albans, Herts, AL1 5SJ, UK
info@panomapress.com
www.panomapress.com

Book design and layout by Neil Coe.

Printed on acid-free paper from managed forests.

ISBN 978-1-784520-78-6

The right of Christopher Babayode to be identified as the author of this work has been asserted in accordance with sections 77 and 78 of the Copyright, Designs and Patents Act 1988.

A CIP catalogue record for this book is available from the British Library.

All rights reserved. No part of this book may be reproduced in any material form (including photocopying or storing in any medium by electronic means and whether or not transiently or incidentally to some other use of this publication) without the written permission of the copyright holder except in accordance with the provisions of the Copyright, Designs and Patents Act 1988. Applications for the copyright holder's written permission to reproduce any part of this publication should be addressed to the publishers.

This book is available online and in bookstores.

Copyright 2015 Christopher Babayode

Dedication

While the stereotypical image of jet-setting pilots and crew is glamorous and a very good advertising tool, the reality has a not so desirable underbelly. An underbelly dealing in real world problems faced by flying crews the world over who sometimes paint on smiles when they would rather not, who stay awake through the night sometimes by choice and sometimes not, who keep unsociable hours and who turn around and do it all again at short notice and increasingly to the dictates of commerce and demanding airline flying schedules. This book is dedicated to them. It is an effort to help them take advantage of knowledge, tools and technology to help make the journey that bit more enjoyable. I hope your Dunlops are dangling!

Acknowledgments

Emily McMorran for her tireless support for me in getting my message out there and for being such an angel.

Petra Lander for the hours spent reading for me and for offering me advice having trodden the path herself.

Mindy, Emma and Charlie at Panoma Press for their guidance, help and expertise in getting this book in print.

Lastly, but not least, to Patricia for all those timely reminders.

PREFACE

When I told my co-workers at the accountancy firm I worked for in 1998 that I was leaving to become a flight attendant, the first thing they all said was, "You can't do that, you know flying is so unhealthy." 17 years later I am still flying and loving it. I've spent enough time flying to know there is a healthy way to fly available to anyone who cares to look for it.

This book is a signpost to healthy flying and jet lag elimination afforded me from the years I've spent in the air. The words from the "you can't do that, it's not healthy" crowd have only served to strengthen my resolve to make flying work for me. One of the lessons I've learned along the way is that success in flying well requires a powerful reason. I found mine and you have to find yours. It could be for the sheer hell of health or more subtly it could be because you know you have so much more to do with your life after flying. It is this kind of drive that will keep you flexible enough to come up with solutions that work. I know it did for me.

It is my intention and aim to spark a conversation among frequent flyers who hunger for something different in the way of jet lag cures, other than the pastiche of cures offered at the moment. We need this kind of conversation because we know frequent flying has more serious consequences other than collecting frequent flyer miles and mileage runs!

CONTENTS

Part I

Part II

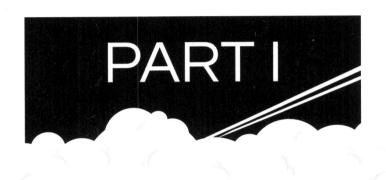

Introduction

Most people believe jet lag is an inevitable part of flying. Truth is, the worst jet lag has to offer can be avoided and is self-inflicted. You can drastically reduce the effect of jet lag by making a small change with a big impact. The change in question is a change in perspective. To date jet lag has been looked at through a very narrow lens, which lends itself to a one-sided type of solution, an ineffective solution at that! All current attempts to cure jet lag stem from this view of the problem. It is a perspective that ignores some of the most obvious and basic observations you could hope to make about the flying experience. The promise of this book is to show you how you can transcend this narrow view, empower yourself and build the solution to any jet lag symptoms or conditions you have no matter how much you travel.

When I speak of a solution for flyers no matter how much you travel, I really mean it. This book is written specifically with frequent flying pilots and cabin crew in mind. They are road warriors who fly long and short–haul with a frequency that defines the flying part of their life as part of their lifestyle.

To be one of these frequent flyers you literally get on a plane at least once a week. You travel all over the world, live out of a suitcase and rack up an average of 10,000 miles a week minimum. You travel so widely that you constantly have to adjust various aspects of your life to suit your travel schedule, from sleep to eating habits to social engagements and so on. You double up on "can't live without items" and pack half of them in your suitcase so you can assemble some type of normality while on the road.

It is this kind of exhausting flying that puts you in a unique category of flyer. It is so unique that when calculating your exposure to cosmic radiation the UK Department of the Environment (DoE) puts you in a class of your own. The DoE describes you as having ionizing radiation exposure as an occupational hazard and requires that records be kept on how much radiation you are exposed to.

Other kinds of challenges that plague this type of most frequent flyer creep up on them in the course of flying year in year out. They go beyond the regular inconveniences infrequent flyers experience like constipation, dry skin and dehydration to include hormone imbalances, thyroid challenges, fertility problems, weight problems, insomnia, narcolepsy, extreme fatigue and other sexual problems. While these health challenges are not unique to flyers, if you fly chances are the flying aspect of your life plays a role in your health picture and probably isn't helping.

One of my past clients came to me because she was about to plan for a family and had heard the horror stories of the persistent fertility problems among cabin crew. She wanted to know what she could do to avoid them. Her main concern was the effect the stress of flying would have on her ability to conceive. We worked on preparation and a detox program for six weeks and not long afterward she was pregnant.

Another crew client had been flying for over 20 years and thought the severe tiredness was just age and job related. We worked together for a month to change that. In that time we made shifts in her understanding of the job and how it affects frequent flyers (you would be surprised how many frequent flyers think any cure occasional flyers use is good for them) and instructed her on simple things she could do to feel different. The instruction was the leverage point that made the difference. By understanding how flying affects you long term, the aim of this book is to help you address any health issues related to your flying lifestyle.

The second part of this book is focused on healthy flying solutions to build vitality in a systematic way that ultimately helps you get a unique perspective on your health. I mention this now because I regularly see flyers who have gone from road warriors to road weary! Vitality is the missing ingredient. Without vitality you are hard pushed to keep going when the going gets tough. If you are the impatient type or you know vitality is the missing ingredient you've been looking for, you can jump over to part two now.

As a frequent flyer for over 17 years I have seen all the approaches to cure jet lag you can imagine. They are all incomplete, superficial, or have no real understanding of the far-reaching effects of what jet lag can do to health long term. If these so-called cures understood the scope of the problem, a one size fits all approach wouldn't be seen as a reasonable solution and the cures they offer would reflect this; they don't.

The pharmaceutical industry is busy trying to get round the FDA so they can drug jet lag out of you[1]. In effect, trying to turn jet lag from an inconvenience into an illness. Supplement companies believe their products are the answer without having a real understanding of the complexity of the challenge. Homeopathic cures suggest approaches that ignore vital aspects of the problem.

While some of these approaches may have some merit for the occasional or vacation flyer, they are not to be reckoned with if you spend your life in the air. Anyone not using pharmaceutical, homeopathic or supplement approaches is usually self-medicating with stimulants, over-the-counter (OTC) medication or recreational drugs or combinations thereof. A 2011 *Business Traveler* magazine article "Power Pills" [2] highlighted a trend in better living through pill popping and it seems frequent flyers of all walks of life have taken this to heart.

If you labor under a heavy transatlantic or global travel schedule while fulfilling a role for your company this book is for you too. Anyone who flies often and needs to arrive ready to perform, without letting the journey get the better of them, can use this book to great benefit. Even if you don't fly so often but suffer terribly with jet lag when you do fly, you too will find this book useful. I will be writing from the perspective of a nutritional therapist and 17 years of cabin crew flying experience. My examples and insights will be taken from that context but they apply to all kinds of flyers most of the time. If you need to stay productive after you have de-planed and flying is a regular part of your function before you perform (whatever that performance may be), read this book.

CHAPTER 1

What Can Frequent Flyers Learn From Savvy Pilots and Crew?

With so much information in the public domain you might ask yourself who is this guy to write a book about jet lag and why focus on pilots and cabin crew? Well, to state the obvious, they are some of the most well-traveled people you will come across. Not only do they travel as far and wide as corporate jet-setters but they also do it with intensity unmatched by any other group of flyers you care to name and I am one of them. There is a saying in personal development circles that if you want to improve yourself don't go with the easy crowd, go where the competition is hard and it will automatically cause you to reach for a higher standard.

As far as intensive, quick turnaround, regular frequent flying goes, pilots and cabin crew set that standard. Don't get me wrong, I'm not saying every pilot and cabin crew member you come across is an expert flyer able to deal with jet lag and the stresses of flying. They are not, but some have mastered parts of the puzzle to suit their lifestyle. It is my job to point out the distinctions they made and show you how to weave them into a system to enable you to reduce and eliminate the worst jet lag has to offer you as a regular flyer. The other reason to stick with me is that having flown for a major airline on short-haul and long-haul fleets for a total of 17 years plus, and practicing nutritional therapy for flyers, I feel I have a genuine worthwhile contribution to make to my flying colleagues and the frequent flying community at large.

I have been there just like you, I have woken up in hotel rooms around the world and not been able to get back to sleep. I have suffered the frustrations, fatigue and stress of being constantly on the road. I know what it's like to fly regularly and run a business at the same time. I know what it's like to have burnout at the beginning of a trip. I know what it's like to go to sleep at night and wake up unrested and unrefreshed and still have to carry on. I know what it's like to lose the will to do anything except retire to the comfort of my bed even when there is much to do. It wasn't until I realized that the slew of available "cures" were energy bankrupting in nature and of limited use to frequent flyers that I knew I had to find another way.

I had to find another way or join the heap of burned-out cabin crew and pilots who no longer enjoyed flying and were stuck in a rut with no zest for life left in them to do anything about it. My moment of clarity was combining my flying experience with my knowledge of nutritional therapy and my job as a crew member. I am a flight attendant first, a nutritional therapist second and a frequent flyer third.

Unlike other books written about jet lag, this one is not just about theory. It is both practical and pragmatic in approach and execution of the solution. It is not a quick fix solution but there are aspects of it that can be applied and benefited from straight away. Its uniqueness is not that this system reinvents the wheel but that it takes knowledge, distinctions and tools from other fields and combines them into a system like none other before it. Making the discoveries that make this solution work are afforded me from the crossroads of a naturopathic nutritional therapy philosophy, an eye for the scientific literature, common sense, key distinctions and experience of having over a decade and a half's worth of flying full-time.

This book is also a tool to enable you to do one thing no other jet lag "cure" can do which is to enable you to build lasting vitality and resilience while you travel. This is as important as any of the other steps to mastering jet lag and healthy flying. Most if not all jet lag remedies assume that you are in good shape for travel from the get go. This is not always the case, and if you are like most people who travel a lot, time is of the essence. So being fit for the road while being on the road complement each other and pay dividends in flying, health, time, productivity and well-being.

Just as an athlete trains for an event, frequent flyers should also train for a life in the air. It is not an additional bunch of things to do, but a decision to make healthy choices that support flying as a regular part of the life of frequent flyers. Just as flying crews go to training school for annual checks throughout their flying careers to make them fit to do the job, all frequent flyers should be in "training" for the road as long as frequent flying is part of their job description.

Why Is a Lifestyle Approach to Jet Lag Necessary?

Jet lag is in fact a lifestyle problem and can only be reasonably solved when approached from a lifestyle perspective. This is a key distinction all cures miss. Up until now the scientific community had led the field with its habit of dissecting aspects of the jet lag experience without accounting for real world knowledge. Theory is fine in a laboratory setting where the variables can be controlled but when so much can change at a moment's notice theory is not always the best approach to a lasting solution.

Before the launch of the Airbus A380 super jumbo and the Boeing 787 there was an ongoing discussion in aviation circles. It centered around which type of aircraft would best suit commercial aviation needs. Would the future favor the A380 with its long range and ability to carry a large number of passengers or the 787 with its combination of range and flexibility to do shorter stop work? Similarly in looking for a healthy solution to jet lag there is a question of which type of "cure" best serves the interest of the frequent flyer. I would like to champion the cause of the long-term sustainable solution over and above the short-term approach prevalent among today's flyers. Here's why:

- Short-term cures don't really work because they focus on battles instead of winning the war

- The long-term proactive approach is more sustainable than the short-term reactive approach

- The increasing rates of burnout and stress we face

- The continuing impact of globalization and technology

Short-term cures don't really work because they focus on battles instead of winning the war

The short-term jet lag cures so popular with most of the flying public don't work. You may find an infrequent flyer here or there saying they do, but if you delve into the definition of what a cure should be (which we do further on in this book) you will see that it falls short.

Short-term cures are not flexible enough to use consistently and ultimately are not as flexible as your flying schedule. The problem is you have to use them every trip. That might have been okay when every trip meant once every couple of months but these days travel frequency has increased so much that it's hard to maintain use of these cures and get the results you once did. If you fly often you are going to run into trouble sooner or later using these half-baked solutions.

More about the specifics of why they don't work later in chapter 2 under the heading "Let's talk about jet lag", but if you are not convinced, ask yourself why there are news headlines almost every other month touting a new jet lag cure; surely if it's been cured successfully once, other cures would be obsolete.

The long-term proactive approach is more sustainable than the short-term reactive approach

Short-term cures, Jedi mind tricks and anything else in between tend to be reactive in the cause of beating jet lag and flying healthily. This is too little too late. Understanding the nature of the challenge will lead you to the conclusion that a lot of the work is actually done and accomplished before you ever step foot on the plane, or if it isn't it should be!

The fact is most people don't think of jet lag until they turn up at the airport or step on the plane. This point was driven home to me when I was discussing jet lag with a business acquaintance of mine. As a regular flyer and globetrotter this was the same view he held. I was shocked; maybe it was because I did so much flying myself that it came as a surprise to me. When I pressed him on this his response was, "I just don't have the time to handle it any other way." The challenge with this is how does he function at his best in business if preparing adequately isn't routine especially as it has the power to affect his productivity?

If flyers don't think of jet lag and how it's going to affect them at the other end until they are on the plane, is it any wonder they turn to short-term crutches to help get them through? What they really need is a long-term strategy once they understand what they are up against. This is part of the problem, flyers don't have a detailed understanding of what they are up against to make informed decisions about what to do and what not to do. Instead they put their hopes in the miracle pill or some other cure that is easily at hand.

The increasing rates of burnout and stress we face

The World Economic Forum 2011 highlighted a trend in the workplace that had been present and is slowly creeping up on people with little comment until now. The title of the talk in the Open Forum was "Burnout... the latest fashion" [1]. While it may have been discussed on a large stage such as the World Economic Forum, burnout impacts everyone because the rate at which we live life has sped up. Frequent flyers are no exception to this phenomenon. There is just too much stimulus out there and we have not yet become adept at filtering it. The results are heavier stress loads and constant changes are the new norm.

I recently read about a celebrity book tour where students repeatedly asked why it wasn't okay to burn the candle at both ends in pursuit of success! It doesn't matter whether it is student life or entrepreneurship, setting oneself up in this manner is not a good foundation for long-term success. If this is the basic idea of what you have to do to be successful and you fly often, it is no wonder short-term quick fixes are the tool of choice to beat jet lag and fly better. Trouble is, all they can do is get you through the current trip in hand while depleting you of vitality, creativity and resourcefulness long term. That is a high price to pay and most people pay it because they don't realize the Faustian bargain they are making at the time.

To make matters worse, the so-called cures flyers turn to are the usual suspects: alcohol, medication, recreational drugs and caffeine. You get the high you need and the low you don't want. The rollercoaster goes on, up and down until you are depleted. Burning out in this fashion is nothing new and has been around forever. The question you have to ask yourself is: is this how I want to continue? Do you want to see your potential pass you by because you failed to use better tools? A long-term approach to jet lag is one of those tools which if used correctly will lift all you do because it builds vitality, which is the most important factor in successful living bar none.

The continuing impact of globalization and technology

As globalization continues to make the world smaller, its impact on our lives is subject to constant change. In business this means there is more competition out there to overcome. In life in general it means there is more information to peruse, use or discard. The magnitude of what we have to deal with to remain ahead grows by the day and if you are standing still it is likely you are going to lose. The change and the opportunity of globalization make for more stress in our lives.

Globalization means we are more connected. Good, bad, useful and useless information travels faster than ever before. It carries the potential to be disruptive. As a frequent flyer this can be quite apparent as you globetrot. It only takes one seemingly unrelated event somewhere else in the world to have ripple effects that could upset you, your travel itinerary or the outcome of your venture. Sometimes it is not even the fact that "something" happened but the awareness and the reaction to that something that change events or become obstacles. A lot of the time we find ourselves in reaction due to this never-ending slew of information helped along by the always on 24/7 technologically connected world. Too much stress leads to overwhelm and paralysis, which isn't good for individual health let alone any goal or travel objectives you may have set out to accomplish.

As globalization and technology are not set to slow down any time soon this is a condition we appear to be stuck with. Yet most frequent flyers still turn to the old staples for relief of jet lag while trying to cope in such conditions. These staples were of limited use in the pre-globalized world and are of even less use with the twin factors of increased demands of travel and the pressures of stress we now routinely deal with in the 21st century. We live in a world where the pressure is unrelenting. If you don't have a strategy to deal with it you are risking it all.

The bottom line is we know the short-term approaches don't work; they've been around forever and only deplete you. Trying something new with a fuller understanding of the challenge and with deeper insight of the problem is a better way forward. If there is one thing I would like to make you aware of it is that up till now all approaches have focused on the short-term view, on things to take for immediate relief, before or after the fact. This might be of use till the next time but if you keep repeating these short-term remedies at the expense of your long-term health you always end up the loser.

Let's make no mistake about it, many have lost this same fight, from those who have overdosed on drugs to those who have substance abuse problems, alcohol problems, sleep deprivation leading to road crashes and worse. If you think long term about the problem of jet lag, you see the necessity of needing vitality to see you through to the end of your frequent flying days; vitality is useful for avoiding all the mishaps above and whatever else you want to apply yourself to in life.

Questions

- What is jet lag to you? What ideas do you have about jet lag?

- How would you have to feel to know you weren't jet lagged?

- What is your general attitude toward your flying schedule? Do you dread it, welcome it, or just get on with it? Why?

CHAPTER 2

Jet Lag Needs A New Conversation

Let's talk about jet lag

Jet lag is destroying health, vitality, relationships and productivity. Jet lag needs a new conversation and it needs it now! Too many flying crew and frequent flyers from all walks of life are paying too high a price for frequent flying. Despite the latest and greatest miracle cures regularly reported in the media, no solution has singularly succeeded in addressing the multi-headed Hydra that is jet lag. Nobody inside or outside the aviation industry is prepared to take this challenge head on. The challenge has been disowned so much that it has been left to vested interests to dictate what jet lag is about by default.

Each party attempting to cure jet lag only sees the problem from a limited perspective, without regard for the other aspects of the problem. While this limited approach may benefit flyers in some small way, it is inadequate and dangerous to the health of frequent flyers in what it disregards. This can be said of all the approaches out there, be they pharmaceutical, homeopathic, supplements, over-the-counter medication, recreational medication, stimulants or dry research theory.

To get to a new conversation about jet lag, what is needed is a 36,000-foot perspective. To bring that perspective into sharp focus there is no better tool than the frequent flyer as a stereotype. Pilots and cabin crew fit that stereotype as will other flyers in the field or industry and beyond, but as I mentioned earlier I am writing this book primarily for the intensive flying community. As such I will tailor most of my observations to them. In order for any approach to be considered a complete cure for jet lag it has to fulfill the following four criteria:

- It must be healthy; there must be no undesirable side effects and no risk of addiction.

- It must be flexible and robust. You should be able to use it every time without plateau.

- It must be portable. You should be able to take your cure with you and administer it yourself without having to wait for the services of a third party.

- It must address all aspects of the flying experience.

Let's go through these criteria one by one

It must be healthy; there must be no undesirable side effects and no risk of addiction.

The most frequent flyers cover a conservative estimate of about 30,000-40,000 miles month in month out. On average they fly once a week. They have minimum rest at the destination and fly back again a day or two later. A cure must be able to withstand this type of flying. Any cure that eventually leads the flyer down the road to ill health is no cure at all. Most of the common cures flyers turn to eventually cause or contribute to chronic and acute health challenges. The favorite safe bet, pharmaceutical grade melatonin, is known to cause complications and has a long list of contraindications and side effects to its name. See the caution table at the website melatonin.com for full details [1]. The U.S. National Institute of Health (NIH), the websites Medicinenet (MNT), Web MD (WMD) and Medscape (MSC) score the list.

The cautions are divided into absolute contraindications, inadvisable contraindications, possible side effects and overdoses. Side effects include problems with autoimmunity, liver and kidney disease, stroke, epilepsy, hormonal effects, reduced sperm counts, lactation problems, disorientation and psychotic symptoms to name a few. Note: If you must use melatonin make sure it comes directly from food sources.

As a flyer if you rely on melatonin each time you jump time zones you are potentially setting yourself up for trouble. You may get away with it in the short term and not notice any adverse effects but hormonal shifts over and above those regulated by the body's normal hormonal output will have a telling effect sooner or later. Our hormones work in concert with each other, supplementing melatonin in this manner risks affecting the entire system. How long can you maintain upsetting the system before adverse symptoms crop up in your health?

It must be flexible and robust. You should be able to use it every time without plateau.

As pharmaceutical melatonin is one of the most widely known/used "cures" for jet lag I will probably refer to it often. From a practical standpoint the use of melatonin by heavy frequent flyers like crew is moot as they would likely overdose by quickly building up a tolerance to it based on their busy flying schedules. Melatonin just isn't robust enough to handle the complexity of their frequent flying. For instance, delays, aircraft changes and repairs to aircraft can change trip outcomes at a moment's notice.

How would someone coordinate taking melatonin long term with all the uncertainty that crops up unannounced in flying? The same goes for those who favor Ambien or Valium and other hypnotics. If flights leave on schedule and there are no delays you can get away with it. But as any regular flyer knows, the chances of delays and disruptions increase the more you fly.

When disruption strikes, those flyers who popped the sleeping pills expecting an uneventful flight are caught short. It becomes an even more dangerous situation if the situation becomes catastrophic and the plane crash-lands or needs to be evacuated quickly. Saving oneself under the influence of a deep drug-induced sleep is not easy nor is it a favorite pastime of the cabin crew charged with executing such evacuations.

Popping pills on flights can sometimes have less serious but still unintended consequences. The story goes that one passenger took a sleeping pill after a delayed takeoff, only to wake up under a pile of blankets in an aircraft hangar, much to the surprise of the cleaning crew sent to prepare the plane for its next flight!

It must be portable. You should be able to take your cure with you and administer it yourself without having to wait for the services of a third party.

One of the watchwords of global travel is self-reliance. It is not fun to be far away from home and at the mercy of someone or something else for your own health or safety. The same applies to jet lag cures. The more control you have, the better chance you have of influencing the outcome.

While networking I have often come across holistic yoga or massage practitioners who say they too help cure flyers of jet lag. It often made me smile, as two scenarios would pop into my head. Did they mean to say that their client had to suffer jet lag on their return journey home before they could beat their way to the said therapist's door to get the cure? Or if that wasn't the case, do they travel with their clients all the time, as you never know you might be jet-lagged on arrival at your destination as much as you could be on arrival back home? In both instances their client would either have had to suffer jet lag for one leg of their journey or find a massage or yoga class at the destination they traveled to.

If the flyer were visiting a familiar location that probably isn't a problem, but if it is a new destination finding a suitable practitioner or therapist can be hit or miss until the destination is familiar. Sometimes flyers (business travelers in particular) have a lot riding on the outcome of trips or first impressions they wish to make. If they are in an unfamiliar location and cannot get their preferred treatment, it is not too unreasonable to suggest that they would show up in less than ideal shape than they could have if they had a portable solution with them all the time.

It must address all aspects of the flying experience.

The loudest voice in the jet lag cure market is the pharmaceutical industry and melatonin crowd. Their argument is that popping a pill or taking melatonin corrects the body clock/helps you sleep/keeps you alert and saves the day. The problem with this straightforward argument is that there are jet lag symptoms that don't respond to pharmaceuticals and melatonin and never will. The challenge is such that there are other aspects of the flying experience that contribute to jet lag that are being ignored. Until these are acknowledged and dealt with there will always be half-cures masquerading as the complete solution.

All current common cures you care to name fail the test by one or more of the above criteria. These criteria matter because of the restrictions the job or trip place on the frequent flyer. Take flying crew for example. Flying crew have to turn up for work at their base station sober on their outbound and return flight. Being under the influence of alcohol is not an option. Indeed there are strict rules and cut-off points surrounding how much alcohol you may consume or have in your bloodstream before reporting for duty.

Crews are expected to turn up for work fully rested so they can be alert and ready in the event of any emergency. If they have challenges with jet lag they may need solutions while they are in some far-flung country as much as they need them on return to base. Waiting to get back home to visit a therapist would only be useful half the time. Pharmaceutical solutions would fail flying crew by the same standards as alcohol mentioned above.

The common cures that are not drugs, stimulants or alcohol fail by only addressing the challenges of jet lag and healthy flying superficially or not at all. Furthermore, no amount of vitamin pills are going to help you cure jet lag no matter how soon you take them after your flight.

Another aspect today's common cures ignore is what I like to term the ecology of jet lag. The interaction of the flyer with the environment of flying plays a role in the experience of jet lag. Most cures tend to take the view that jet lag is done to us. There is some truth to this notion, however if there was greater understanding of the ecology of the flying environment among flyers some cures would be seen for what they really are – a waste of time.

Instead most of the attention is paid to remedying jet lag after the flight. The peddlers of jet lag cures focus on short-term cures that don't stand the test of time and take frequent flyers deeper into energy bankruptcy and vitality deficits. The drugs, over-the-counter medicines, off-label prescriptions or other stimulants eat deep into energy reserves leaving the flyer less able to recover over time. Their only respite is to take time off away from flying for total rest and recuperation but that is not always an option, nor does it actively rebuild the lost resources and deep energy reserves by itself.

Frequent flyers from all walks of life have to answer the basic question, "Do you want a truly healthy cure to jet lag or are you content to bundle through with half-cures that lead you down the path of health problems and burnout?"

The current solutions lead to adrenal fatigue and hormonal bankruptcy. If you get it that hormones and the endocrine system are important to your health you know that this is too high a price to pay. As hormones run the show in many areas of our lives, including sex drive, reproduction, menopause, andropause, sleep, emotional well-being and immunity, relying on "cures" that upset the hormonal system is asking for trouble at some point in life. Some research studies have found pilots and cabin crew to have a higher incidence of prostate, skin and breast cancers, which are all hormone related. Another piece of research by the University of Durham [2] demonstrated that long-haul stewardesses have higher saliva cortisol levels than short-haul stewardesses (deranged cortisol levels are known to be signs of stress). The implication from this research is that raised stress hormones and frequent long-haul flying are correlated.

Here comes the difficult part of this new conversation about jet lag. If you ask the average person on the street what the cure for jet lag is they will most likely say melatonin. If you repeat that question and answer to a seasoned traveler it might get mixed reviews. Why do you think that is? One answer is that there is no unanimous agreement about what jet lag is. Yes there are a bunch of symptoms that are shared but flyers don't limit themselves to these. For some it is the inability to sleep on the plane or away from home. For others it is being awake and asleep at the wrong times, while others complain mostly about the total lack of energy or motivation to do anything. For some of them melatonin may be of some benefit but that does not mean it is right for every flyer.

As a supplement melatonin is known for helping you nod off to sleep by encouraging sleep onset but if it is sleep quality rather than sleep quantity that is the issue melatonin may have little benefit. That is why a flyer can take melatonin for jet lag and get good results to start with only to see the results taper off or have no effect as they continue to use it. Supplementing melatonin is not the answer for everyone. A better basic understanding of the production of melatonin will provide better ways to manage problems that arise from its absence and sleep-related challenges. See the "Rhythms" step in part two of this book for specifics on how to do this elegantly.

When looking at the marketplace's attempts to cure jet lag I see three main players: the pharmaceutical, supplement industry, and the homeopathic approach. These approaches all differ in how they see the problem. This in itself is part of the problem. There is no watertight theory or understanding of what jet lag is and therefore there is no uniform approach that gets it right every time. At best, depending on the flyer, some of the approaches work some of the time. Some will disagree with me about the definition of jet lag but it is usually defined as a desynchronized body clock. I take issue with that definition on two fronts.

Firstly, if jet lag is just about the body clock, why is it that when melatonin, a known regulator of the body clock, is used the results flyers get are not consistent? If the problem was desynchronized body clocks and melatonin cures that, everyone should get cured of jet lag every time. As we know, this is not the case, it is hit and miss.

Secondly, melatonin may have a reputation as a super antioxidant and a hormone but those credentials do nothing when it comes to the dehydration, increased exposure to cosmic radiation or the crushing fatigue that can come with jet lag. The correct view in my opinion is that the body clock is one of the reference points with which to gauge the challenge flying presents but it is not the only one. The definition of jet lag circumscribed by the activity of the body clock is too limiting and misses out other important aspects of the problem.

To make this point another way, let's look at jet lag as an acute and chronic form of stress. After all, if you break down how the body responds to jet lag, this not a bad way of looking at it. The symptoms are a stress on the body and they can be chronic and acute: fatigue, headaches, insomnia, a lack of motivation, a lack of energy and sleep deprivation are a few. When you look at it this way, ask yourself: if I am fatigued, have a headache, am dehydrated or lacking motivation would I reach for melatonin? You might if you had insomnia or were sleep deprived but if your other symptoms persisted you would still need to remedy the situation. As such there cannot be a single drug, supplement or homeopathic remedy that works in all these areas to effect a cure. It would be nice if there were but it just isn't the case.

We Need a New Definition of Jet Lag

To attempt to find a cure that is sustainable and at the same time healthy we need a broader definition of jet lag that simultaneously incorporates all the different aspects of the problem. The working model that suits our purposes is:

Jet lag is a challenge to the body's normal mode of functioning in a *compromised environment*, which upsets patterns, reference points, energy and the equilibrium of our being.

This definition makes the distinction about the environment we are dealing with by labeling it a compromised one. This is very important as it speaks to the nature of one of the principles we must grapple with in order to find a lasting solution. When I say it upsets patterns I am referring in part to the function of the body clock but it is not in the limited way most drugs or substances used like drugs do. Reference points and equilibrium refer to our biochemistry and our physiology and will become clearer the more we develop the principles of healthy flying in this book. Armed with a new definition of what jet lag is we can begin to look at the challenges it poses as well as some of the contributing challenges surrounding the problem which would help us find better solutions.

So while there are many who relate to jet lag from the challenges of getting to sleep and issues of the body clock, there are those who do not. If you ask a flight attendant what jet lag is you may be surprised to hear them mention anything but sleep and the body clock; some will even say they don't get jet lag. For frequent flyers like flight attendants and pilots the signs and symptoms of jet lag can look quite different. Flying crews are more likely to name stress, biliousness, forgetfulness, clumsiness, hormonal issues, weight problems, fatigue or issues of sleep quality before naming sleep per se.

Common Cures for Jet Lag Dismiss the Environment

It might seem novel to focus on the flying environment but throughout the history of mankind adapting to or conquering an environment is something we have always done to ensure our survival. It is no different in the air. To fly better means mastering the flying environment of the cabin and recognizing that it is quite different in the air than when on the ground.

What I am speaking about is the ability of our species to adapt to a set of conditions in order to survive (in this context I mean to thrive on arrival). When man decided to explore the oceans he invented diving gear that allowed him to explore the depths. When he decided to explore space he invented a different kind of kit that allowed him to go where no man has gone before. When he attempts to tread the highest landmass on the planet he at least takes oxygen with him. In every case where humans have thrived or conquered an environment we have shown our adaptability by taking our environment or elements of it with us. Thriving while flying is the same. It means understanding the environment properly, planning accordingly and executing according to the knowledge we have about the environment.

At the moment this is not how people fly. They board a plane, behave as if they were on land and think their normal behavior in a foreign environment has nothing to do with how well they are on arrival. Moreover, the jet lag cures they reach for have no understanding of the flying environment to effect a decent cure.

The nature of the flying environment makes it important to solving jet lag. Yet common cures ignore it totally by concentrating on the period before the flyer goes into the flying environment, the period afterward or not at all. Alcohol and drug misuse may be the exception to the rule (if you count them as cures) but it is impossible to drink or drug yourself week in week out as a frequent flyer and still perform at your best.

The flying environment in more detail:

- Less than ideal oxygen
- Lacks moisture and is dehydrating
- Encourages positive ions
- Spreads noise pollution
- Fosters a disordered sense of time and place

You might take it for granted that the flying environment is pressurized to the altitude of a small mountain (between 6,000 to 8,000 feet) but it has consequences for the flying experience you are subjected to. In trying to compensate for the discrepancies created by flying at altitude, air is bled off the engines and fed back into the cabin. At altitude that air is quite dry and some of that dryness is reflected in the cabin air. This lack of humidity in the cabin is drying to all flyers and has other physiological consequences. It increases the amount of dehydration taking place in the cabin and within the flyers themselves. It leads to an increase of static in the cabin and also an increase of positive ions in the cabin air. These are all a source of stress to the body.

The human body is used to more humidity, less static and a more even balance between positive and negative ions in the air. No amount of melatonin, Ambien, Nuvigil, No Jet Lag homeopathic pills or B vitamin laden drinks does anything to address this.

I'll say it again: jet lag is a type of stress, extreme stress. Stress is a theme running through all challenges jet lag poses to the body and there are multiple factors involved. The flying environment is one of the two major ones we have to deal with. The flying environment is stressful because it is hypobaric in nature. This means there is low air pressure and low oxygen content in the air. While this in itself is not outright harmful it does mean the body has to work harder to function normally. It is also noted that the effects of this environment can be worse for flyers who are stressed or ill.

Other often overlooked stressors of the flying environment are noise and vibration. Even with the advent of technology planes are still noisy. While we may get accustomed to it, the noise is still stressful to our physiology. Exposing yourself to higher decibels over long periods of time is not something we are accustomed to and this takes its toll on our central nervous system. Along with noise, aircraft engines cause vibration which is distributed all over the aircraft. We absorb this stress every time we fly and it may be one of the least recognized stressors we face when flying.

Stress caused by a disordered sense of time and place comes about through the fact that you appear to be traveling so slowly while you are in fact going fast. This is disconcerting to the delicate mechanism that looks after our sense of balance. Flying also takes us out of our natural earthly rhythm. The Earth itself gives rise to waves that resonate from within its core out into space. The upper limit of that resonating chamber is the Schumann resonance, which is sometimes seen as the luminous white line around the Earth from space. Flying disrupts our connection with this rhythm.

The Schumann resonance rhythm is part of our natural environment on land and has similarities to the alpha brainwave frequency in the human brain; my feeling is that its absence/disruption when flying is akin to being lost and contributes to the disorientation felt after flying. In fact, research by the California Institute for Human Science (CIHS) is now indicating that connecting to the Earth restores the natural electrical balance within our bodies [3]. If this is the case you can imagine how stressed the body is after a 10-hour flight without being able to make that connection.

If you break jet lag down on this basis how many current jet lag "cures" do you know that address all of these factors adequately? This is just the beginning. We haven't factored in the health of the individual, the effects of alcohol and caffeine available when flying, food and snacks available or the stress the flyers board the plane with. The reason this and all these factors are important is that in the final analysis these stressors lead to quicker disruption in proper functioning of the physiology. A build-up of toxins and acidity accompanies this. Over acidity in flyers is bad for flying and bad for health. All current cures fail to address this.

Are You Jet Lagged or Jet Stressed?

Another distinction to make is that there are actually what I would call two kinds of jet lag. One is the experience the infrequent flyer has after a trip and the other is the experience of the frequent flyer. It is important to know the difference so you can choose the appropriate types of tools for the type of flyer you are. The difference in the type of flyer you are is the difference in someone with an acute or chronic condition. At the moment, all flyers get lumped together by the symptom pictures they display. The infrequent flyers have the acute picture while the regular flyers may have some acute symptoms but the majority of their symptoms are chronic in nature. When I explain it I like to say that infrequent flyers get jet-lagged and frequent flyers get jet-stressed.

Jet lag is an experience any flyer can have while jet stress is a process, a process entered into the more hours you fly. As a process it follows a particular pathway. Unfortunately this pathway is one of deterioration marked by a decline if nothing is done to change things. I have seen too many of my flying colleagues battle with this kind of deterioration not to mention it specifically here. Typically it starts out with the stress picture they are unable to deal with and involves one or some of the following: an energy picture, a hormonal picture, an immunity picture and an immunity system breakdown picture. These pictures are related and to a certain extent don't always follow a chronological order; whatever the case, they all impact health and sometimes with fatal consequences.

The gravest picture is the immunity system breakdown picture that might show up as a cancer for example, while an intermediate step might be adrenal fatigue or other hormonal or fertility issues. Recognizing which of these pictures a flyer has as a jet-lagged frequent flyer allows them to trace their steps in the opposite direction to build vitality instead of deteriorating further.

The point I am making here is that while the infrequent flyer has more of a chance to recover from their symptoms, given that they don't fly so often, the frequent flyer is locked into a commitment with an unfavorable outcome due to the amount of flying they tend to do. The experience of flying infrequently yields a very different effect from the experience of continually repeating the feat over a period of time. If nothing is done to remedy the situation the frequent flyer obliterates their health and immunity. Yet if you look at the marketplace the kinds of cures available don't make this distinction and peddle the same kind of remedies to all types of flyers.

A Stress Model for Jet Lag

In trying to create a successful outcome in the management of our particular type of jet lag, or should I say jet stress, we would do well to piggyback on the best understanding of stress we have to date. Some of the tools devised to help understand stress in the medical sciences are useful to us as frequent flyers.

Dr. Hans Selye's General Adaptation Syndrome model (GAS) is ideal in this respect. It can be summarized as follows: we have a normal level of resistance we operate from. It handles the day-to-day stresses we encounter without much deviation or expenditure of resources on our part. If a stressful event over and above this were to happen it would cause us to go into an ALARM response. If the stressful event were not remedied we would then go to a RESISTANCE stage (typically marked by the body using more resources to try and remedy the situation but lowering overall immunity). If that failed or more stress was applied we would then go into the EXHAUSTION stage. The three stages chart going from a state of resisting the stress to being unable to do so. The power to preserve our immunity is the desired outcome here as it is the ultimate protector.

As a frequent flyer you are stuck in the resistance stage or variations of it. As time passes by it becomes harder to get out of this stage and back to "normal" immunity without concerted effort. The longer you keep flying, the more you trigger the resistance stage. The more you trigger the resistance stage, the greater drain on your vitality. If not checked this leads to the exhaustion stage.

Having defined jet lag as stress and knowing what stress can do to our health, any jet lag cure worth its name ultimately has to not only eliminate stress but also help build vitality. This is the litmus test for any cure. At the moment all common cures fail. Vitality is the ultimate antidote to stress. With enough vitality you have deeper pockets to handle the stress that comes your way. With enough vitality you will bounce back better and stronger. As the saying goes, health is not the absence of disease but the presence of vitality. Having redefined what jet lag is, looking at the principles that underlie it is in order.

Questions

- Are you jet lagged or jet stressed?

- How did you arrive at your answer?

- How much do you unwittingly contribute to your jet lagged or jet stressed state?

CHAPTER 3

The Determinants of Jet Lag

If someone told you it was your fault you have jet lag I bet you would disagree. While it is not entirely true, there is some truth about it. One of the simplest reasons most flyers get jet lag is that they don't know what they should stop doing in order to fly better. There are many factors and symptoms that make up a jet lag experience but at their core they boil down to a handful. As well as not knowing what not to do there are snake oil salesmen in different guises shouting about their latest cure. Include pharmaceutical companies, inventors and supplement companies in that group. They peddle selective jet lag theory and limited experiences as proof.

If that is not bad enough, it's the assumption that everyone else experiences jet lag the same way that stifles a worthy solution. The scientists research more and more minute areas of human physiology as if jet lag was strictly a mechanistic phenomenon. The middlemen on the other hand just get potions with some vague health benefits and hope it brings some kind of relief to flyers. The inventors invent gadgets without acknowledging any other factors about jet lag.

To know what to stop doing means you have an inkling that what you are doing has undesirable effects. This alone is not enough to solve the problem though. A closer look at a frequent flyer's journey and the environments they find themselves in hold valuable keys to unlocking the potential of a lasting solution. If flyers got out of their own way and used the foundation laid out below as their guide they would do a lot better and carry the keys to a better flying experience with them whenever they flew.

The Three Principle Determinants of Jet Lag

The basis of our approach to understanding healthy flying, jet lag and its challenges are Environment, Entrainment and Acclimatization. I think of these as principles, as every step we use to create a solution to jet lag has its roots in one of these principles. Flyers who successfully experience any kind of healthy relief from jet lag use one or some of these steps whether they know it or not. By healthy relief I mean they do no harm to themselves in the immediate or long-term period. Having said that, there is a difference between accidentally being able to produce a result and knowing how all the variables stack up, to enable you to reproduce it every time you fly. What we are trying to accomplish here is mastery. It comes when you have an unshakeable context with which to view and manage all the "moving parts" of the problem.

At the center of this principled approach is the flyer; he or she boards the plane in a particular state, in mind and in body. The default starting point for every flyer is some sort of stress; it could be physiological, circumstantial or mental. American Express Business Traveler Survey 2007 claims 43% of travelers are stressed out before they get to the airport [1].

The jet lag principles are about restoring balance to this distressed state using multiple approaches at all stages of travel and even when you are not flying. Once this is achieved the goal then becomes how to sustain this long term and build vitality along the way. I hasten to add that while the last two sentences may have sounded a bit cumbersome, in practice they are not. Think of it like this: as someone living in the 21st century you know you have to take more care of your health among all the other things you have to accomplish. With the P.H.A.R.E. Well System, which is our methodology of dealing with jet lag, you are able to kill two birds with one stone.

My training in nutritional therapy is with a basis in naturopathy. It is the lens with which I look at the problem of jet lag and frequent flying. The strong point of naturopathy in my opinion is that it strives to stay in keeping with the Hippocratic oath of "do no harm." This is very important especially when you look at the side effects and dangers some of the touted cures for jet lag have.

Not doing any harm now or down the line is what makes the P.H.A.R.E. Well System safe and unique among all other offerings available for jet lag. These principles and the approach we are describing are aimed at doing no harm and charting a pathway to even better wellness, normally cut short or disrupted by frequent flying and the stressful events of modern day living. Restoring balance is at the heart of the matter, as is the ability to thrive despite all the odds against you.

If I could say it any better, I would say that as far as jet lag is concerned, flyers are so alienated from natural health factors in their environments that when they fly the out-of-sync-ness manifests glaringly as jet lag. The Environment, Entrainment and Acclimatization principles take root in our natural healthy states of being. This novel view of jet lag and the natural healthy environment asks questions of the current accepted knowledge regarding air travel. It also offers clues to making course corrections that benefit all travelers in terms of a jet lag free flying experience.

Environment

Apologies to James Carville whose campaign slogan for the re-election of Bill Clinton was, "It's The Economy, Stupid." In our case, "It's The Environment, Stupid." The stressors of the cabin environment on the plane are relatively influential based on the internal environment the flyers board the plane with (i.e. their internal terrain). In this sense we are dealing with two separate sides of the same coin. The fact is they both influence each other, but the greater leverage to create influence in the direction of health lies in taking control of the internal terrain environment. This is the first task of every frequent flyer wanting a healthful solution. This is why it is important for every flyer to know what they need to stop doing to gain control over their internal environment.

We constantly manipulate our internal environment based on many factors of our lives: what we eat, what we think, how active or inactive we are, how much sleep we have and other things. In order to maintain our survival and functionality the body has developed a system of balance that keeps all these factors in check so they do not threaten life via our biochemistry. This mechanism is the homeostatic balance of the body.

In correctly functioning human physiology the homeostatic balance is kept within a particular range. The body, the blood, cells and organs have ranges they must stay within in order to perform optimally, and the intelligence of the body is scrupulous in maintaining these norms because derangement can lead to drastic deterioration in health and even death. Flying upsets some of these norms and the body does its best to rectify them. It does its best to maintain the optimum environment whatever the instance. We must support the body in this effort as much as possible and give it more of the tools and resources it needs to do this important job.

The general consensus is that the human body thrives in an overall environment that is tipped slightly toward the alkaline side of the pH scale. The pH scale is a tool used to measure how acidic or alkaline a solution or environment is, using its hydrogen and hydroxyl ions (they carry a negative and positive charge respectively). There are organs that are predominantly acidic or specifically create acidic conditions in order to function, but the blood for instance prefers the alkaline side of the scale. As the blood gets everywhere in the body, this will be our marker when it comes to our ability to buffer acidity. Managing the pH of the body is important as it affects the body's homeostasis.

pH Scale

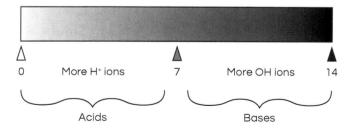

0   More H⁺ ions   7   More OH ions   14

Acids   Bases

Diagram 1: pH scale

Altitude changes the environment by depriving us of the protective dense layer of oxygen we are used to at sea level. The oxygen we breathe is used to fuel our metabolism including the digestive and respiratory systems. The less than ideal supply of oxygen at altitude means we start to accumulate more toxins, potentially making us more acidic.

The foods and beverages served on board create even more acidity and hit our bodies with a triple whammy. Regardless of this assault, the homeostatic mechanism kicks in and regulates the various aspects of our metabolism so we can continue without much trouble. If you are lucky, at worst your urine turns a darker shade of yellow signifying that you are more dehydrated.

The environment is such an important factor to consider in the equation of healthy flying that it would be wrong to discuss it without mentioning the trend of installing Wi-Fi capability on planes. As far as I know, the trend of installing Wi-Fi on planes started around 2009 in the United States. It was seen as an extra stream of income for the airlines that had been hit hard by the economic downturn in 2008. If you took a hard look at the competitive airline business it is easy to see that this extra stream of income would be an attractive proposition. However, it is also plain to see from a healthy flying perspective that it is a bad decision. Gadget emission and Wi-Fi signals in a confined space add to the woes of flyers.

Cosmic radiation at altitude in the presence of less oxygen is able to do more damage as noted. Adding Wi-Fi radio waves into that environment is making things worse not better. Anything we can do to lower the exposure of flyers to all types of ionizing and non-ionizing radiation is a step in the right direction. We all like convenience and want to be entertained on flights but the introduction of Wi-Fi is the equivalent of smoking on flights of the 1970s, only much worse! The traveling public doesn't know what this costs in terms of their health over the long term. Just because the cabin environment looks the same at takeoff, cruise and landing doesn't mean it is. Airlines need to look at the bigger picture and educate their flyers instead of going for the easy revenue option.

In summary, recognizing that the flying environment is harsh and less than optimal allows you to plan ahead and take steps to counter its ill effects. In practice most of these steps can be taken care of as part of a lifestyle approach. The first step is recognizing the environment is different and treating it with that respect in mind.

Entrainment

The Environment is the larger vehicle for the other two principles of a healthy jet lag solution. The environment we live in naturally imparts us with the habit of entrainment. What I mean by this is that we are naturally entrained to the Earth's rhythms. On the surface this happens superficially with day turning to night and vice versa. At a deeper level the Earth's core radiates a field reaching out through the layers of the Earth and out into space. The outer portion of this field's edge is known as the Schumann resonance. It is otherwise called the Earth's brainwave. As human beings who have always lived on this Earth we have always been in tune with this resonating field. While not totally accepted in certain scientific circles there is reason to believe the influence of this resonating wave is essential and beneficial to human health. For instance, the human brain is said to resonate in similar ranges when it is in the first octave of the alpha brainwave frequency.

As Earthlings we used to live in harmony with this wave pattern until we started creating different patterns with technology and moving further way from nature. Being close to nature is one way to stay in tune with this entraining habit. As such it is actually the absence of this entraining habit at altitude that combines with other factors and leads to jet lag.

The entrainment habit is such a strong trait in humans that it has even been observed in the menstruation cycles of women living together. It is known as the McClintock Effect [2]. Although the pheromone theory of how it works is criticized, the lunar influence effect is yet to be disproven. The naysayers may say it is unproven, but if the lunar effect can move the tides on the oceans and the bodies of water in us I think it is a bit too hasty to dismiss it out of hand just yet. To put it poetically, we live in sympathy with the Earth that gave us life.

The specifics of the research from the California Institute for Human Science (CIHS) (see Jet Lag Needs a New Conversation) suggest that the human body is dynamically checking its reference to the Earth every 90 seconds. Our break from this very important reference is so stressful it also contributes to jet lag. As the human race has continually widened the gap between itself and nature, using the seductive artifice of all manner of technology, our out-of-sync-ness is becoming more evident.

The normal patterns of life are disrupted on many levels with frequent regularity every day of our lives. The Industrial Revolution meant more people moved away from land to the cities to find employment, thus cutting the connections they had with nature and agrarian lifestyles. The light bulb turned night into day altering natural sleep and wake cycles. Modern lifestyles mean people see exercise and the outdoors as optional instead of a regular part of living. All this disharmony increases the stress we face and further keeps us out of sync with our environment and ourselves.

It is against this backdrop that most flyers board a plane. Unrested, out of sync and with low levels of chronic stress of one order or another. When translated to the physical body this stress is very real. It disrupts the body's optimal rate of metabolism. This can manifest in many ways: elevated blood pressure, shallow breathing and tenseness. When this happens it's important to remember that tensing up restricts blood flow all over the body. This is the last thing you want to do; the net effect of stress in the physical is the production of more acids in the body, which is exactly what you don't want. More acids equal more toxins, more toxins lays the ground for you to get to know jet lag better.

Much is made of the body clock's role in jet lag. Its role is highlighted here in the Entrainment principle. The P.H.A.R.E Well approach departs from the common notion that the body clock is the be-all of jet lag. For our purposes the body clock is an approximation for the time value we put on our day-to-day living experience.

We all conduct our affairs based on the 24-hour clock and yet science tells us our bodies run on a clock of 24 hours 11 minutes with a variation of plus or minus 16 minutes. The research points out that light exposure is the key to resetting the clock to run closer to 24 hours. I take this to mean there is room for flexibility and it can be made to suit you once you understand your daily rhythms.

The idea that your body clock (time) is flexible and can be manipulated will be alien to left-brained flyers; to them it defies logic, however we have all experienced those times when time expanded or contracted independent of the 24-hour clock. Body clock research explains this concept better by saying that the hard-wired clock of 24 hours and 11 minutes is re-aligned by our natural exposure to light by the day and night cycles. We can duplicate this effect within our travel schedules with a little know-how. Becoming adept at doing this is something that every competent jet lag free frequent flyer does.

The tools used to train your body clock to do your bidding will be discussed later on in this book but for now we can group them all under the heading of Zeitgebers. What are Zeitgebers? Taken from German it means time givers. Anything you can use to give your body a sense of what time it is from your external environment is a Zeitgeber for our purposes. I say for our purposes because in the scientific literature Zeitgebers refer specifically to certain cues.

As creatures of habit we can use our habits to suggest circumstances that create desired outcomes, like telling our body what time we want it to be through habitual actions. When you look at the body clock in this manner it becomes one of many tools to use to get the outcome of a jet lag free trip. Becoming adept at what cues work best for you is a matter of trial and error but once you notice the ones you are influenced by you can set your schedule up to take them into account.

Acclimatization

If Entrainment is about balancing your internal environment, Acclimatization is about getting in sync with your external environment so you can slot right into the time zone you find yourself in. Getting acclimated is more about the things you can do in and about your new environment that allow you to adjust quicker. As the saying goes, when in Rome do as the Romans do – this is a good rule of thumb to abide by. It is the difference between landing on the west coast of the United States from Europe and going out and about in daylight to adjust, rather than going to bed right away because your body is still clocked to night time in Europe. Acclimatization is in many respects a lighter form of Entrainment but it does not deal with the deep-seated drivers that control the many functions that are unbalanced from a long journey like Zeitgebers do.

The great thing about acclimatizing correctly is that there are many "tools" in the environment you can call upon to reinforce the idea of acclimatization upon your body. It is important to do this, as with both acclimatization and entrainment you have to work with the tools until your body takes to the entrainment or acclimatizing effect. Having a choice of tools to use to acclimatize allows you to do this dynamically.

Now that we have our three principles in place, the next chapter explains the six steps that have their roots in these principles. This is the actual P.H.A.R.E. Well System and what it stands for. If it is not obvious by now, the idea is to take the steps on board in the knowledge of where they came from and how they may be manipulated to suit your specific flying outcomes and lifestyle.

Questions

- How long do your trips tend to be?

- Are you able to get on to local time easily? If yes, what do you do specifically; if not, can any of the principles above help?

- Are you able to acclimatize quickly once you return home?

- What routines do you have for yourself away from and at home?

CHAPTER 4

The P.H.A.R.E. Well System of Jet Lag Elimination and Prevention

I waited in vain for the words "healthy flying" to become fashionable. While healthy flying may sound like an oxymoron it is a real possibility if the right perspective of flying is taken. I have been trying to give and explain the correct perspective one needs to accomplish this up to this point. By now you should be fully aware that this idea of healthy flying is only valid if you the flyer decide to take more care of yourself when flying.

This cure is one brought about by the handiwork of you the flyer regardless of whatever else may happen. It works because as a flyer you choose to take the long-term view of the challenges of flying while everyone else looks for short-term solutions. It works because you choose to take on board the best practices and habits of frequent flyers the world over who fly well and arrive well.

The six steps presented here are the steps to flying well under any circumstances. You can learn, absorb and incorporate them into your lifestyle so they become second nature. The most important thing to do to get long-term results is to practice them as regularly as you fly and outside of flying. Conquering jet lag and flying healthily is a process not an event.

The six steps to master in your flying lifestyle:

- Protection
- Hydration
- Acclimatization
- Rhythms
- Environments
- Wellness

Protection

To the untutored eye the environment of the plane stays the same as when you boarded the plane. As the plane gains altitude, its systems adjust the atmospheric pressure in the plane similar to that found on a small mountain. This is done because the plane will ascend to heights of about 36,000 feet where oxygen is scarce making it harder to breathe naturally. Adjusting the plane's environment to that of a small mountain about 8,000 feet high is a form of protection for all flyers. As the flight progresses the air gets drier and the cabin builds up with positive acidifying ions. These cause you to feel stuffy and lethargic. Changes are afoot in your physiology that lay the ground for jet lag. We all need protection from these and the cascade of effects flying sets in motion. That is why protection is the number one step in mastering healthy flying and beating jet lag at its roots.

One other significant factor flyers need protection from is ionizing radiation. There is more cosmic radiation (with the potential to ionize) bombarding the plane at altitude. More of it gets in the cabin at altitude so it too adds to the threat. As flyers and frequent flyers we need protection from the external and internal environments generated from flying. I know there is an ongoing debate about ionizing radiation and the damage or lack of proof of the damage it does to human health, so let's look at the facts.

The undisputed threat of ionizing radiation lies in the fact that it can cause damage at the DNA level and cause genes to function in ways that are harmful to health. Ionizing radiation is a fact of life and a natural phenomenon in the world we live in. It should not be feared for its own sake and it is a challenge to health that does have a natural solution. Tapping into that solution is a priority every flyer should undertake to stay healthy regardless of how much they travel.

Up until his death, Dr. John W. Gofman was considered the foremost expert in the field of the effects of ionizing radiation on human health. Gofman was also an expert witness in court cases against the nuclear and radiation industries. Dr. Gofman's 1982 book titled *Radiation & Human Health* suggests that small doses of ionizing radiation are cumulative and could prove to be dangerous to health over time. This is the single fact every frequent flyer should be aware of: the more you fly, the more exposure you risk. With awareness comes the desire to do something about it, this is a good thing.

More recently I came across work catalogued by the National Academy of Sciences (NAS) on ionizing radiation, specifically low-level ionizing radiation. The work comes under the heading BEIR which stands for Biological Effects of Ionizing Radiation. The work is a collaboration of the top scientists from the National Academy of Sciences. It is worth noting that contribution to the NAS is by invitation only. The work of Gofman and the scientists at the NAS clearly acknowledges the risk ionizing radiation poses to human health. The question to ask is what can you do as a flyer to minimize the risk and stay protected any time you fly?

The correct answer is what we've always done about ionizing radiation! As I said above, radiation has been around forever and people living in areas of naturally high radioactivity have survived it. Once you acknowledge the problem has a solution within your reach all you need to do is work out the steps you need to take to protect yourself. The challenge with taking these steps is that the fear of the topic is stopping the widespread discussion of the problem in its tracks. No proper discussion of the problem equals no solution equals nothing gets done and flyers' health suffers.

Being a naturopathic nutritional therapist, the most complete framework I've come across on how to deal with ionizing radiation comes from my training in naturopathic philosophy. The core idea is about protecting yourself through building immunity. In fact the U.S. Environment and Protection Agency (EPA) supports this in principle. This is demonstrated via the below diagram.

Protection Basics

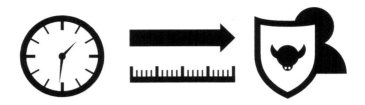

Diagram 2: Based on EPA protection basics

The diagram introduces the idea that time, distance and shielding are the precepts in reducing harmful exposure. In plain English it is saying that the less time you spend in the presence of radiation, the further you are away from the source and the more shielding you can have between you and the source, the better. It must be said that while the EPA diagram demonstrates the solution in a somewhat superficial manner, the kind of solution we are constructing starts with building protection from the ground up in the physiology.

Protecting the body and its organs through building immunity is how you make sure you have adequate shielding. You could do this by building a lead bunker or wearing lead shorts but there are practical obstacles to taking them with you every time you fly! The smart way to protect yourself is to do it through your diet. There are foods you can incorporate into your diet that fortify and protect your cellular structures from ionizing radiation. There are also foods you can habitually ingest that bind with ionizing radiation metabolites and safely move them out of the body. While it is definitely a good idea to start eating some of these foods, understanding why this is a valuable tool increases your chances of success manifold. It boils down to your body having the intelligence to want to protect itself – you just have to help it along the way.

In summary, making sure you are protected when you fly is everything. Even with the brand new generation of planes leaving Airbus and Boeing none of them can change the fact that the flying environment is a hostile place to be for extended periods of time. Building immunity on an ongoing basis is the best way forward.

Hydration

Low humidity in the aircraft cabin is a problem all flyers face which leads to dehydration and constipation. Yellow urine is one of the first telltale signs this is taking place in the body. Truth is the environment created at altitude disrupts the entire body's physiology. Staying hydrated matters because of hydration's knock-on effect on other systems of the body. In terms of proper functioning, hydration is a basic currency. As you become more dehydrated, the body's fluids become more concentrated with toxins, which weakens the body's electrical potential.

Many processes of the body rely on electrical impulses. Water plus the negatively and positively charged elements of our diets can increase or decrease the amount of electricity available to us. Together they encourage the conduction of impulses that run various functions. The saying goes that life was electrical way before it became mechanical and biochemical. As such, the impact dehydration has on health and biochemical functioning of the body is not to be overlooked.

The delicate balance of fluids has always been one of the most important ways we maintain the function of electricity in the body to support proper functioning. Maintaining homeostasis is challenging to the body in conditions of dehydration. The net result of dehydration is that the body does its best to preserve essential functions but the build-up of acids and toxins makes it harder. Reversing the drying effects of flying that happen every time you fly is easily overcome by staying hydrated. Some beverages offered on flights do a better job than others; water should be the number one choice. Even though supplies of water are limited on a plane, you can still come out ahead if you pay attention to the water you drink habitually and if you understand the principles of hydration.

We know water is made up of hydrogen and oxygen in a particular ratio. What is interesting about this are the properties of hydrogen. Hydrogen, the first element on the periodic table, is one of the most prevalent elements in the universe. It is found throughout space and this is why it is interesting to us as frequent flyers. One of the natural properties of hydrogen is its ability to neutralize the effects of ionizing radiation.

This observation is not lost on the scientists at NASA. When a theoretical manned space mission to Mars was planned, one of the obstacles was the large amount of cosmic radiation the manned flight would have to deal with. There was also the possibility of solar storms from the sun with large amounts of ionizing radiation frying the mission.

The scientists set up models to protect the astronauts. The first was to have the crew retreat to a bunker in the heart of the spacecraft and the second method was the build and integrity of the construction of the spacecraft as protection. In the latter it was found that a material made with a hydrogen polymer was able to stop alpha radiation particles from penetrating the spacecraft and it slowed the journey of beta radiation particles. Alpha particles of radiation are potentially more damaging to the physiology than beta particles.

The end result was less radiation breached the spacecraft hull. To date NASA continues to fund research of this polymer and uses it in the spacecraft it builds. It looks certain to find uses in other fields away from space travel.

The takeaway for us is hydrogen's ability to reduce the tendency to absorb ionizing radiation, but this is only available to us if we remain optimally hydrated. Tools to do this can be found in the type of diet we choose, the quality of water we consume habitually, and in some cases the supplements we have at our disposal.

Acclimatization

As habits you practice rather than a principle that drives habits, acclimatization practices are all the things you do whenever you arrive at a place to get your body working in tune with the new environment you find yourself in. To make the distinction and separate acclimatization from entrainment habits, acclimatization habits include things like limiting the amount of sunlight you expose yourself to on arrival because you want to stay on your departure country time. Eating a predominantly carbohydrate rich or protein rich meal to encourage alertness or foster a relaxed state to encourage sleep, or limiting or increasing social activity. These and various other habits can make a difference in how quickly you get on to local time.

Knowing when and how to acclimatize may change depending on your schedule and what you want to get done. If travel takes you all over the globe it will differ depending on which part of the globe you find yourself in. The most important thing to note about acclimatization is that it responds to multiple inputs. As human beings we are responding to multiple stimuli all the time. At some level we choose to act on some stimuli while ignoring others. To make acclimatizing an effective tool and get the best result we sometimes have to repeat a stimulus or set of stimuli until it takes.

Rhythms

Rhythms is shorthand for biological rhythms but because there is so much more involved it is a bit of a misnomer. Rather than looking at rhythms as just dealing with the body clock, the P.H.A.R.E. Well System looks at broad hormonal balance as part of good housekeeping habits that are so important to flyer health long term. Included in hormonal imbalances is anything from reproductive challenges to thyroid functioning, weight gain and adrenal fatigue. The good news is that the hormonal system works off a feedback system that means their proper function and balances are all related. When you have an understanding of your own hormones you can begin to work holistically to balance them in sustainable ways without the aid of pharmaceuticals.

The encouragement from the pharmaceutical industry to use drugs to alter the functioning of the biological clock is misplaced when you look at how interconnected its functions are to other aspects of health. Long-term flyers who have used pharmaceutical interventions for jet lag often find themselves with related hormonal issues.

Flying so much means differing levels of exposure to daylight, one of the most potent controllers of hormone activity in the body. Besides daylight, diet can also be used effectively to get similar results particularly where melatonin is concerned. With an eye on health and sustainability of solution diet is the better choice over pharmaceutical intervention, which can be disruptive on the whole system.

Mastering your rhythms without the aid of pharmaceuticals should be the aim of every frequent flyer. Any other means is not robust enough to do it long term without affecting the biofeedback mechanism all hormones work off. Often when a client presents their case in clinic, pharmaceutical hormonal intervention is part of the challenge. In part this is because they suppress the natural rhythms of the body.

Environments

Environment mastery involves practices to influence the effects the flying environment has on your body. Ultimately it starts with mastering the internal environment of your biochemistry. In reality it is only really about the internal environment, but because flyers are ignorant of the effects of the flying environment, it is necessary to understand both the cabin at altitude and the individual's biochemistry separately. Flyers look at the journey they take as the sole culprit in any experience of jet lag they may have. They don't understand that habit and lifestyle factors outside flying contribute to the severity of their symptoms.

In order for flyers to stop being victims of jet lag it is a must that they understand lifestyle effects on jet lag and build new practices into their life. So instead of a short-term view of jet lag as a flight-by-flight occurrence, we are advocating the view of jet lag and healthy flying as requiring lifestyle tools as much as any other kind of tool.

Key to mastering your internal environment is knowing the importance of the pH scale as mentioned earlier (see Determinants of Jet Lag); it goes along with being able to master homeostasis. Food thoughts and emotions we indulge in produce biochemical effects that are acid or alkaline in nature. Environment mastery is about staying predominantly on the right side of the pH scale, the alkaline side. To get the benefit of this tool you only need a simple understanding of acid/alkaline balance and the willingness to add more alkalizing practices into your life.

I am sorry if I sound like a broken record on this point but when I fly I constantly get asked, "How can I beat jet lag right now?" Well, the answer is if you haven't looked after your internal environment any other tools I can offer you will be of limited use. To hit the ground running on arrival, flyers who mean business have to avoid most of the standard fare offered to them by airlines and perhaps become more vociferous in asking for better options.

Some would argue that there is a place in society for alcohol, sugar-laden drinks and caffeine abuse but an aircraft cabin isn't it. I know this won't be popular with all those flyers and airlines that provide and consume this stuff or see it as an indulgent treat but this is the truth.

They pollute your inner terrain at a time when it is already handicapped by the flying environment.

The fact that airlines serve caffeine laden beverages and alcohol and offer a thinly disguised warning for you to consume them in moderation is a clue. They don't want to tell you not to use them outright because they know how unpopular that would be. After all, we've been sold on the glamorous, luxurious and indulgent view of flying for a long time now.

Wellness

Wellness tools are any tools that promote the cultivation of vitality – generally and specifically. Anyone who exercises on a regular basis automatically has this advantage. They have more energy and are more vibrant. Unfortunately not all flyers recognize that this advantage is available to them or that it is important.

A recent survey conducted by a business travel provider asked frequent business travelers to list in order of preference things they felt were necessary for a good business trip. Fitness facilities came last on the list, far behind Wi-Fi connectivity and late checkout facilities! This survey speaks volumes about the attitudes toward health among the majority of business and frequent flyers. Truth is, while everyone is keenly performance driven, not taking the time to nurture health to drive sustainable performance leads to burnout and less than stellar results.

A recent Bloomberg TV news story estimated jet lag costs the U.S. economy $70 billion in lost productivity annually [1]. I would argue that the United States is a prime example of the flyer burnout phenomenon a focus on wellness can address. The United States has the most complex airspace in the world today. It has four time zones with nine climate zones on the mainland alone. Negotiating the skies on business trips in the U.S. can be an arduous process.

The changeable weather these time and climate zones provides plus the sheer distances within U.S. borders means that business travelers experience fatigue and flyer burnout faster than most other frequent flyers around the globe. The cost of burnout can be mitigated with an emphasis on traveler health; slowly but surely it seems corporate America is beginning to see efficiencies in this area can pay big dividends.

Physical exercise should be at the core of a health and wellness routine for all flyers and all flyers should have a routine. Exercise is not optional, it is mandatory for flyers who want to stay at the top of their game. The exercise choices to consider should include aerobic, resistance and restorative practices. They all have specific benefits flyers should learn to appreciate.

One of the great things about flying in the 21st century is that we have better technology. Technological advances mean there are tools flyers can use to fly better, recover faster and perform better. The best thing about these new technologies is that they are all portable which means you get instant feedback. This is what you need when there is so much variety as it allows you to monitor your progress and course-correct if need be. While flyers tend to be early adopters of technology in the gadget field, it is about time they took advantage of technology that helps them fly better (see the "Protection" step in part two).

The wellness aspect of this program starts with the idea that training for the journey should be an ongoing endeavor. The more resilient you are, the better you will deal with the challenges that pop up along the way. Being physically fit is a precursor to feeling better and better performance in any field of endeavor.

The P.H.A.R.E. Well solution does what it says on the tin: it enables you to fare well in all respects. It means you sacrifice nothing in terms of your health and well-being. No one wants to spend a lifetime flying only to find themselves burned out, but many do. While short-term approaches might give you instant short-lived results, it comes at a price you can't pay indefinitely. This is where a holistic approach like ours comes into its own. The P.H.A.R.E. Well solution puts you in the driver's seat for the entire ride – at home, on the plane and at your destination. It takes note of and caters to the three constants every frequent flyer faces.

The Plane

Can you use all or part of your chosen solution on the plane? Can it travel with you conveniently? Portability is important. Take the number one obstacle on the plane, a pressurized environment which encourages dehydration and acidification. What does your cure have in its arsenal to combat this and its side effects?

Your Destination

Can part of or your entire cure help you adjust quickly to your destination so you can get your outcomes with minimum disruption? Can your solution support you in doing your best work? Again, as you are far from home the tools to accomplish this have to be portable to be of long-term value.

Home

Do you pick supportive solutions that work well with your lifestyle at home? Home life is full of distractions and disruptions of our own and others' making. How do you avoid them? For example, if you know you have to pay attention to your sleep but know sleeping in is not an option for you, maybe going to bed early is. Making sure you understand the rhythm of your lifestyle will allow you to plan practices that support healthy flying. Your right type of solution should be able to slot in alongside whatever lifestyle you have as a matter of priority.

Using a solution that works well across these three constants should be your aim as you will be moving between them continually. The trick is to move your solution between all three without any hiccups or disruptions. What I'm really pointing at is if you use the common cures for jet lag – caffeine, alcohol and OTC medication – can you see yourself using them in each of these settings with no negative consequences?

It is my hope that some of the information in these six steps sounds familiar; maybe you have been using them without knowing how they stack up together to build a robust system you can use. The questions that follow are aimed at helping you focus on how to bring your knowledge to the forefront so you can consolidate it and commit it to unconscious competence.

While I have explained the P.H.A.R.E. Well System, if you are stuck on its relevance to you and your travel plans the next chapter should give you an idea of what you face when you go out there to catch that next flight. I'm not saying you don't know but if you stop and think about it you might just get another 36,000-foot view.

Questions

- Which of the six steps do you use now?

- What resources do you use to implement the steps you use?

- Which steps do you find the hardest to implement? Why?

- How can you devise a plan to overcome these challenges?

CHAPTER 5

Why the P.H.A.R.E. Well System is an Idea Whose Time Has Come for Frequent Flyers

A Timely Reality Check

I think it was Brian Tracy who once said most people are in a race they are completely unaware of. That race has been named and framed by Thomas L. Friedman in his book *The World Is Flat* to be globalization. The pace of life fueled by globalization means competition is greater than ever before. Opportunities are briefer than before because it is now a crowded marketplace and you face competition you didn't know existed. These are the paraphrased words of Joel Roberts, an expert at distilling the essence of the dynamic world we now live in. This means resourcefulness is at a premium. On a worldwide playing field with stress in pursuit at every turn there is no greater resource than personal health.

The sheer volume of information coming at us tests our resilience and health. In this era of accelerated globalization, information moves more freely. We have at our disposal a wealth of information which is growing exponentially. This means circumstances and decisions can change at a moment's notice and with them outcomes that affect you. Because information travels faster than before, change is a constant now. Being able to adapt to change is a skill everyone needs to acquire; doing so without stress and hassle makes for better productivity and superior performance. The consequence of not adapting could be dangerous for you, your livelihood and the things you care about. As a frequent flyer always on the move, building that resilience muscle is now part of the game plan, and part of that involves a strong foundation of personal health.

Technology as a communications tool has its pluses but it also has a downside. It has run amok and is close to controlling people's lives. It is a disruptor as much as an enabler. Business people and frequent flyers in particular tend to be early adopters of technology and therefore are predisposed to both the good and the bad it has to offer.

Good is being able to communicate in a timely fashion from different parts of the world to make things happen. Bad is being so glued to your mobile device that you have withdrawal symptoms if you are deprived of your screen for 24 hours. Worse is the effect it has on the way we live. One notable example is Delayed Sleep Phase Syndrome (DSPS). This is where using mobile phones, laptops and iPads, which emit blue light, interrupt your body's natural melatonin pattern.

On a totally different tack, the redeeming thing about the way technology dominates our lives is that it causes us to hunger after an intensity of experience we would not otherwise get to feel: the value of the real face-to-face interaction, which is not to be taken for granted.

Presence is where it's at, there is nothing like being there yourself. Presence of mind, of person and thought are what is required to do your best work and enjoy the best moments. If you think presence is overrated, look at the costs of not being present. It is said that U.S. Secretary of State John F. Dulles lamented that maybe the Suez Canal crisis of the 1950s would not have escalated as it did if he had not had to tend the affair in the state of jet lag from all the flying he had to do. We see more statesmen and women fluffing their lines and making mistakes on the international stage because of the rigorous international travel schedules they have to maintain.

Do you remember a certain airline advertisement of the 1990s where the conniving big wigs at head office summon a subordinate from a regional office for an early meeting? They expect him to arrive on the red eye flight, disoriented, jet lagged and tired; he doesn't. Instead he takes a better flight and arrives present, rested and ready to face them. Business knows the value of being present to make a good impression or decision because it can be costly otherwise. In our personal lives it matters even more; after all, it is our personal lives that hold the real juice of our life. Who wants to travel halfway around the world for a family get-together only to be too tired to participate with family you rarely get to see on a regular basis?

We are All Global Citizens Now

Some flyers think they can get away with ignoring what goes on in the world around them. They ask, "What has globalization got to do with me?" For starters the world in which globalization is taking place is the same world as your workspace. Politics, industry, environment and weather factors that affect globalization also affect you. Even if they don't affect you directly it doesn't mean you won't feel the impact. We live in such times that these many variables increase change and uncertainty we are exposed to. May I remind you that this trend is not set to change any time soon. It is important to pay attention for this reason alone. The best we can do is to find certainty to help us manage the uncertainty that surrounds us.

In this job of flying and increasingly in the global economy, opportunities for situations to interrupt us are at an all-time high. If you don't have a coping mechanism and are repeatedly exposed to these kinds of stresses, eventually it wears on your health and burnout is not far behind. You need to pay attention so you can take evasive action if need be. The ultimate coping mechanism is looking after your health to withstand the stress and whatever the journey brings. The P.H.A.R.E. Well system is designed to add a surplus of vitality to your life so you can meet these challenges and thrive above and beyond them. It is the ultimate adaptogen.

U.S. Secretary of State Hillary Clinton

Secretary of State Hillary Clinton broke the record for visiting more countries than any other U.S. secretary of state by visiting 112 countries and clocking up in excess of 800,000 miles. Four months after she resigned from her position, Clinton quipped she was still jet lagged.

Source: The Presidential Approach to Jet Lag http://maphappy.org/2014/04/presidential-approach-jet-lag/

Hurricane Sandy, erupting volcanos in Norway, political unrest in Thailand, the Gulf Wars, airline takeovers, strikes, and the consolidation of the airline industry are all examples of political, industrial and environmental events that have affected frequent flyers in the recent past. These events have had the effect of displacing flyers and wreaking havoc on many aspects of their lives from the personal to the economical, the financial, health and well-being. This is a constant all frequent flyers live with. With so much happening all the time and so much potential for things to go wrong in such a complex endeavor as frequent flying, the impact is magnified when it does go wrong. Stress can seem overwhelming with any one of the aforementioned incidents let alone the many other things happening at once. On top of this scenario, factor in the immediate stress jet lag generates by itself.

It's Time To Upgrade

Airlines and other bodies in authority haven't stopped giving out the same dated advice and flyers still follow it expecting different results. Way back, airlines' recommendations were: drink plenty of water, get enough sleep and keep your mind active. That may have been sufficient then, when flying was less stressful. Now flying and the growth of the global economy make it a totally different environment to work and fly in and yet the advice has remained the same. A quick look at the history of aviation sums up what I mean.

After 1945 the commercial airline industry really took off. Advances came in the shape of the D.H. Comet, the first jet liner aircraft to be put into commercial airline use, followed by the Russian Tupolev Tu-104. This was followed by the Boeing 707, which is acknowledged as the first commercially viable jet engine plane. It is also seen as the plane that set new standards for safety and comfort at the time. The 707 established Boeing as the foremost aircraft manufacturer in the world with the succession of other aircraft in the 7x7 range: the 727, 737, 747 and so on. In 1984 Airbus introduced the A320 to the world as the first commercially viable fly-by-wire aircraft.

The airline industry has continued to grow with contributions from both Boeing and Airbus in the shape of the 787 and the A380. Over time most of the focus has been on making better planes, the focus has been on what you might call the hardware. The software has remained relatively the same; by this I mean the seating, comfort, the entertainment, the food etc. Just as aircraft have been upgraded through time, airlines need to upgrade the advice and tools (flyer health advice) they give flyers to meet the demands of a world where people fly more often and more intensely. It's time to upgrade the software!

Shying away from updating and giving specific flyer health advice is the source of some of the problems for flyers. Take flying crew for example: they get flying fatigue, have poor attendance records, health issues, high stress levels and have high levels of alcohol abuse and my guess is that there are similar patterns in workforces with business flyers too. These challenges are not well comprehended by the human resources departments. In airlines, it takes a performance-managing trip with an in-charge crew member for a manager to get a feel for what the job is really like. Frequent flying fatigue is not a made-up notion, it is a real day-to-day experience flyers have. Leaving flyers to their own devices in terms of how they manage fatigue is not a wise choice if their function affects others, be it in business or working in a group with some accountability.

Fear of Consequences

We now know more about cosmic radiation and its effects on the body than we did before. Frequent flyers are exposed to higher doses of radiation. Depending on who you speak to, this has led to higher instances of cancer among crew particularly breast, skin and prostate cancers. While it is impossible to prove or disprove that frequent flying causes cancer, there are those who would love to hold airlines or the aviation industry responsible. We know this much from the class action cases brought against airlines when deep vein thrombosis (DVT) surfaced as a health concern for flyers. It is my belief that this kind of hypocrisy makes it harder to have a frank conversation about conditions on the aircraft that might prevent flyers having a healthier flight.

Unlike some quarters I believe the airlines should not bear sole responsibility for looking after the welfare of flyers, or crew for that matter. The flyers themselves should make it an active part of their duty to themselves. At the same time, an airline's position of relative power should encourage them to lead this type of conversation instead of ignoring it. That way all aspects of the problem are out in the open and are discussed with no hidden agenda. The way things are at the moment individuals blame airlines and airlines expect individuals to take responsibility regardless of the conditions they (the airlines) put in place.

Jet lag needs this new conversation, a conversation between all parties involved. It should include the aviation industry itself, the crew who fly and manage the planes, the industry regulators, the passengers and corporate clients and the travel industry. Without a new conversation, the industry and the public are bound to continue along the road of less than optimal productivity. Airlines risk leaving their passengers in the hands of tired crew, with fatal consequences. In business, corporations risk sending their best men and women for the job only to have them arrive too tired to perform at their best, or make the favorable impression needed to open new channels of business. The industry regulators suffer by being labeled incompetent for not putting safeguards in place and thus ruin their reputations. No one wants to invest or work in an industry deemed unsafe. More importantly and to the point of this chapter, flyers need this conversation because they are the ones out there at the sharp end risking life and limb to get the job done.

We are Responsible for Our Own Health

The background to this much-needed conversation about jet lag starts with an individual's responsibility to themselves. When dealing with such a large number of flyers it cannot be any other way. Getting flyers to take personal responsibility for their flying health may be an uphill struggle for various reasons but it is paramount. It is time to ditch the old view that flying is glamorous to start with. It may have been once upon a time but this is no longer the case. It is a hazard to health especially if no remedial steps are taken to counter its ill effects. A complete system like the P.H.A.R.E. Well System helps flyers take responsibility. As it is under the control of the individual flyer it is the perfect tool. It covers the flying environment, the health of the flyer and helps the flyer build that much-needed vitality and well-being with supporting practices. This is important; no one flies for the sake of it, flying is a means to an end.

U.S. Secretary of State Henry Kissinger

Henry Kissinger, former National Security Advisor and Secretary of State, was aware of the effects and dangers of jet lag. Recalling his negotiations with North Vietnamese diplomat Le Duc Tho, Kissinger noted: "[w]hen I went directly from a transatlantic flight into talks, I found I was on the verge of losing my temper at North Vietnamese insolence – nearly falling into their trap by playing the role they had assigned to me. From then on I never began a negotiation immediately after a long flight."

Source: Dan Caldwell & William Hocking, "Jet Lag: A Neglected Problem of Modern Diplomacy?" *The Hague Journal of Diplomacy* 9.3 (2014): 281-295

At the moment flyers are left with a mixed bag of "cures." These cures make the classic mistake of borrowing energy from the body's emergency store without the ability to pay it back. If you fly regularly and are always on the go you don't have time for cures like this. You need to have a dependable source of energy without having to dip into your emergency fight or flight reserves.

In my opinion, cures that exhaust flyers are some of the most dangerous ones available. As well as using up emergency reserves and unbalancing hormone levels, they push the body to points where ill health results. One of the telltale signs in the body of this is disordered cortisol production. Cortisol shows you how much stress the body is under. The danger is that when cortisol production is chronically low or excessive adrenal fatigue and immune system disorders are not far behind.

It might be at this point that the unfortunate flyer turns to traditional healthcare avenues. The problem is these places are overburdened with demand anyway. Depending where in the world he or she may be, or if they have private healthcare, it's a question of pay to play. No cash, no care. That is a risk most flyers take. We can reverse it by doing all we can within our power not to become a victim of the status quo. It starts with understanding our own health and becoming responsible in its care.

A Warped Understanding of the Problem

Jet lag as defined by the most scientific standard is seen as a condition of a disordered body clock which can be rectified if science can unlock the mysteries of the body clock. To that end the focus of discussion surrounding jet lag has been limited to understanding and enquiring into the functions of the body clock at the exclusion of looking at any other lines of enquiry. The definition of jet lag is circumscribed by the body clock understanding of it. This is a major error in the way we look at the problem before we even attempt to find ways to cure it.

Our awareness of what the problem is affects the resources we bring to the efforts we make to find a solution. Before we move on I want to make it clear that the body clock does play a part in the jet lag picture but it is not the only factor in the equation. So far, looking at the body clock as the solution has meant a neglect of other factors of equal importance. Research institutes are fond of telling us about the latest discoveries they have made concerning the body clock and as time goes by they are getting good at amassing a great many interesting facts about the body clock without getting any nearer to solving the problem. The narrow focus on the body clock hinders finding a sustainable solution.

Broadly speaking, making the body clock the sole focus of effort to find a solution does two things. It concentrates too much effort on the body clock part of the equation with little to show for it while at the same time neglecting a more inclusive approach to solving the problem. You can rightly make the accusation often leveled at science which is that its attention to detail misses the bigger picture. This is exactly what is happening here.

The attention concentrated on body clock cures is disproportionate to the focus on the other factors. The middlemen push the use of Viagra as a jet lag cure and many frequent flyers self-prescribe with off-label medicines such as amphetamines and barbiturates. One pharmaceutical company tried to change jet lag from an inconvenience to a disease treatable with its soon to expire patented product. Others have spent time and money developing jet lag glasses and photon showers which all look exclusively at attacking the problem from the angle of the body clock. Jet lag is so much more. It involves the biochemistry which the body clock is directly responsible for, but you would find it hard to relate dehydration, hypoxia or absorbed radiation and other effects to the body clock.

Dehydration, hypoxia and cosmic radiation are features of the external environment created each time we fly. They are ever present, barely perceptible and affect every flyer.

The narrow focus on the body clock does not account for these factors. If a cure were found to immediately reset the body clock each time you arrived at your destination, it would have no material effect on these factors, so the body clock equation is a partial solution at best. The body clock obsession is skewing the argument and these other factors are not getting the attention they deserve. To give them equal footing would provide a more balanced approach to solving the problem at every level while including all the factors that make up the problem.

The narrow focus on the body clock is also evident to me when I discuss flying with crew and pilots. Typically they don't relate to the idea that they get jet lagged, indeed they say, "I don't get jet lag." They say this because they are referring to the definition of jet lag, which means they have an out-of-sync body clock that plays havoc with their sleeping pattern. On further questioning, when I ask about their energy, concerns about cosmic radiation, hydration or weight issues, they all express frustration. For frequent flyers these concerns all play into a greater picture of what jet lag is and can mean.

To try and talk about jet lag without looking at all the factors is a non-starter especially for frequent flyers. Let me explain how with a simple example recently in the media. It is becoming increasingly common for athletes to collapse from dehydration while on the field of play. These athletes are of the highest caliber and they are demonstrating the damage acute dehydration can do to the body. Chronic dehydration over time is equally as damaging.

Chronic dehydration is what frequent flyers put up with when flying frequently over time. No body clock cure is ever going to address dehydration in a meaningful way for flyers yet it is part of the jet lag picture. Dehydration has been shown to be detrimental on the metabolism of the body; it has also been shown to decrease productivity by as much as 25% according to some studies. This is a situation any employer sending their representative into the world of business would like to see the back of. Who wants to have someone with a quarter of their productive capacity removed represent them? No one, particularly airlines who send pilots and crew to fly the planes and be safety guardians on flights or companies looking to close business deals.

I have already mentioned the advice from the U.S. EPA department and the findings of the National Academy of Sciences BEIR files. The body clock has no answers to the challenges or dangers these institutes highlight. Flying is a stuffy affair, as mentioned there is less oxygen in the air. Less oxygen at altitude affects every metabolic system adversely in the human body. The body clock solution will do nothing for this part of the problem.

From the examples I've given, can you see how the ideas about what jet lag is in practice can inform the argument of a reasonable way to define what jet lag really is? Yes it might be that body clock sleep pattern disruption is a major symptom but it is not the only symptom, moreover its cure does nothing for the bigger picture. Putting the body clock part of the equation into its proper context will be an element of the discussion in part two of this book.

Dry Jet Lag Theory Trumps Jet Lag Reality

It might seem to some that my argument is based on an anti-science platform but this couldn't be further from the truth. Using science to understand the world we live in has brought us many benefits and it continues to do so for all our benefit. While science has its usefulness, when it comes to jet lag and healthy flying I think it is a case of not being able to see the wood for the trees, or should I say the trees for the wood in this instance. The exploration of the minutest detail is complicating the route to a holistic sustainable cure for jet lag. It is the way of science to be theoretical before it moves to proving its ideas in the field. The scientific approach to jet lag suffers from this mindset. Scientists and chronobiologists who are undoubtedly experts in their fields base their observation in the sterile environment of the laboratory and not the fluid moving reality in the field. They are cut off from the field of play where and when it really matters.

One of the more reputable jet lag diet cures is the Argonne Institute Anti Jet Lag Diet [1]. It appreciates that changing biochemistry influences how we feel after a flight and the institute designed a diet to manipulate the body's biochemistry. The diet is also time specific on when to use the various tools of the diet. In an ideal world this could be a great solution but the truth is it is too rigid. As a flyer looking at the diet with many other things vying for my attention, the first thing that comes to mind is how am I going to find time to implement all these steps when some of the factors in my travel itinerary are always beyond my control? Or at least beyond my control enough to make adhering to the diet a struggle. How am I going to do this week in week out? While the diet might work to a degree, you can't argue that it is healthful. In my opinion, as good as the diet may have been it was conceived in isolation from the field of play. This makes it a good idea but a lousy tool in practice. It is jet lag theory versus jet lag reality.

The Ehret and Scanlon jet lag book *Overcoming Jet Lag*, reputedly issued to traveling United States State Department employees, also suffers from some of these mistakes. In particular it recommends the use of a group of substances known as methylated xanthines. These substances include the caffeine and caffeine-like substances in tea, coffee and chocolate. As a really frequent flyer how are you supposed to perpetually consume copious amounts of caffeine without getting strung out on caffeine highs and exhausting your adrenal glands or depleting minerals from your body? The Scanlon book suggests adjusting two or three days out from the intended day of travel; for frequent flyers who arrive back home and are off again in as little as three days' time this is impossible to maintain.

Soviet Communist Party Leader Leonid Brezhnev

Soviet Leader Leonid Brezhnev on a visit to the United States noted he was wearing two watches – one set on Moscow time and the other on Washington time. Brezhnev noted that the two watches enabled him to keep track of his body rhythms, but he went on to indicate that he was not sure whether he was seven hours ahead or behind. At Camp David two nights later Brezhnev's disjointed comments suggested that he was still affected by jet lag.

Source: Dan Caldwell & William Hocking, "Jet Lag: A Neglected Problem of Modern Diplomacy?" *The Hague Journal of Diplomacy* 9.3 (2014): 281-295

I once heard a very good piece of advice for going into business; it was a warning not to take business advice from books written from a purely scholarly perspective. This is the same thing those who are getting the most attention regarding jet lag and flying are peddling. As well meaning as they are and as well founded as their ideas may be, not living the life of a frequent flyer severely hampers their views. More often than not they are only seeing a part of the picture of jet lag their expertise relates to. No one piece trumps the others when it comes to finding a solution that is healthy, sustainable and vitality building.

Time and time again you see people with expertise in a particular field, be it science, well-being modalities, nutrition or herbal medicine, give what on the surface may be valid and useful advice. They may have even gone as far as working with flyers, yet they do not make the distinction about different types of flyers nor do they understand the need to. One person may love flying while another does it even though it makes them feel quite uncomfortable. Do you think if you looked at the biochemistry of both of these types of flyers it would tell a different story? Do you think if they took medication supposed to help or cure jet lag it would have a different reaction than normal? Two people can be jet lagged yet have different symptoms. Experts not making simple distinctions like this claim to have the answer to jet lag. Powerful distinctions like this are important to make when dealing with a variety of people who regularly fly in the alien environment that is the aircraft cabin.

The net effect of the jet lag theorists winning over the reality of jet lag is a bunch of tools that do nothing for the plight of the frequent flyer. At best they may help some minority of flyers if the expertise caters to the symptoms they suffer. In areas where the so-called cure depends on a physical visit to the expert, the flyer is forever locked into having to depend on that expert or enduring the jet lag until they can get around to visiting the expert for the cure. If you fly week in week out this is not an ideal situation to be in. Something you can manage yourself is a much better option. With so many variables flexibility is the name of the game.

Incomplete Solutions

You cannot look through the current mix of news media without coming across one article after another tantalizing the reader with the dream of a cure for jet lag. What they all have in common is a distinct lack of imagination in deciphering the root cause of the problem and addressing it.

All of these cures focus squarely on a narrow range of the problem to the detriment of all flyers and with no hope of really being able to conjure up a solution worth shouting about. I have leveled the accusation that science is theoretical in its approach to jet lag and all available cures take their cue from this approach. What makes these "cures" incomplete is the misunderstanding of the problem in its entirety, right from the conception of what it is, down to the best way to attack it with the surest chance of success. If you take a closer look, the solutions offered barely fit the problem. They constantly produce ever diminishing returns until it impinges on health and gives way to more serious health challenges. In a society with an ever increasing pace of life and accompanying stress this is the worst approach possible.

The first thing all or most of these attempts at a cure have in common is that they lead to exhaustion by over taxing the sympathetic nervous system. The Sympathetic Nervous System (SNS) is the part of the Autonomous Nervous System (ANS) which controls our fight or flight response. In its original conception this system was meant to get us out of danger in emergencies. Relying on this system as the default mechanism to deal with jet lag has many problems. The flip side of the SNS is the Parasympathetic Nervous System (PNS); it is the foil of the SNS, it balances its activity and restores balance back to the body. It is in charge of restoring homeostasis when the body goes out of balance. The most common approaches to jet lag cause this imbalance by stimulation.

All caffeine-based stimulants fall into this category. Tea, coffee and amphetamines all act on the sympathetic nervous system causing excitement and ramping up of the fight or flight mechanism. Doing this on a continual basis, flight after flight, exhausts the energy and eventually the adaptive response of the body to deal with emergencies. Depleting the body's resources like this brings greater levels of fatigue and exhaustion at deeper levels. This leads to the general feeling of exhaustion and specifically the situation where people wake up after a night's sleep but do not feel refreshed. They easily accumulate sleep debt and a vicious cycle ensues.

The habit of borrowing energy from our reserves is endemic to frequent flyers of all walks of life. The Facebook group Flight Attendants asked flight attendants how they managed to stay awake during the night sector flights: 85% of the 146 answers said they drank coffee to stay awake. What is more troubling is that no one seems to see anything wrong with this practice. There is a case to be made for the occasional use of caffeine but to make it fully effective the habitual use of it must be stopped. Using it routinely takes away from the desired effect when you use it judiciously. To put this information in context refer back to the work of Dr. Selye's stress model the General Adaptation Syndrome (GAS) (in Jet Lag Needs A New Conversation) which establishes the model of the biological stress response.

The use of stimulants like caffeine triggers this first stage of the GAS system, the SNS is under fire and causes the production of cortisol which tells the body it is in a state of stress. Using this system too often when it is supposed to be reserved for emergencies weakens it and draws from a store of energy that should only be used in emergencies. When it is used inconsiderately like this it can lead to lowered immunity when other stressors come into play with the immune system. In my clinic working with frequent flyers it leads to adrenal exhaustion, which is the gateway to many other health challenges. It is important to remember that cortisol and adrenaline are hormones. Hormones work together in concert. When the actions of some are disordered they can compromise the function of the entire endocrine system.

It is important to make several points. Triggering reserve energy of the body on a regular basis is not the best way to get energy while on the go all the time. It is inefficient, costly and counterproductive. Energy debt quickly ensues and catching up to get ahead becomes harder as more caffeine is used. Also, global travel and the shifts the body clock has to make to shift time zones is energy intensive. Coping with different amounts of light exposure when traveling east or west makes things worse and restorative sleep can become elusive. Sleep onset, which is controlled by melatonin, is in turn influenced by natural and artificial light exposure. It is easy to see how you might get into a vicious cycle, all the while depleting precious energy reserves with no way of replacing them.

Besides frequent flyers demonstrating immune system weakness, medical statistics show there is a pandemic of autoimmune disease. The American Autoimmune Related Disease Association (AARDA) report (see the Why Flying Has Changed chapter) estimates autoimmune disease is the number two cause of chronic disease. Where autoimmune disease used to make up 20% of cases presented to GPs about 20 years ago, it is now thought that they make up

80% of cases. The increase is not down to a single factor; some causative factors include environmental toxins we are all exposed to as our world has become more toxic and polluted. Living in a more toxic world is something we all have to take into account as flyers and as citizens.

Stress is marked in the body by inefficient function and in the cellular structures it is typically marked by an acidic condition of the cellular environment. Stress accumulated externally or internally from any source is an obstacle to the body in an alien flying environment and a contributor to jet lag. Acid emotions, thoughts and body make for a toxic internal environment that is capable of upsetting the balance of the body, perpetuating the vicious cycle. To break this cycle it is important to get out of the habit of using short-term solutions, which have negative impact long term.

A real tragedy of incomplete jet lag solutions is that none of them actively build vitality. Building vitality while living out of a suitcase is no mean feat and is not to be underestimated. You need energy while on the road and travel is physically intensive. The right kind of exercise will help while the wrong kind will deplete you further. Bringing this mindset to your attitude toward exercise and recuperation can help you become more matter of fact about sticking to a regular program. Other jet lag cures settle for ridding you of some symptoms of jet lag without looking at the bigger health picture. The assumption they make is that you are healthy to fly. The lifestyle the flyer has and their health is a less important factor to them.

Just as health is not the absence of disease, settling for the absence of symptoms as a solution to jet lag would only be half the problem solved; you must have vitality. If you have ever gotten off a plane after a long trip you know what I mean. You have that sinking feeling in your gut that drags you down and makes you feel awful. You are still buzzing unpleasantly from being vibrated at speed in the upper parts of the Earth's atmosphere, and now you have to go face some cranky customs officer! These symptoms and situations are draining and can be overwhelming long term. While you somehow dredge up the strength to carry on, the journey grinds the vitality out of you and you never get off scot-free. Whether it is the physical discomfort of flying, the stress of the journey process or the anticipation of what lies ahead, they always exact a toll on you and your well-being.

The vitality sapped by flying needs to be replaced on an ongoing basis. This is especially important the more you fly. A lifestyle-based answer to the question of building vitality is the only reasonable solution because being on the road so much doesn't leave a lot of spare time for much else. Even though flying conditions have gotten much better with the advance of technology they are still unable to completely alleviate the effects the harsh inflight conditions have on human physiology. Until inflight conditions are no longer a factor, frequent flyers will always have to learn to adapt in order to overcome their less desirable effects.

Adapting to build vitality on a regular basis is the preparation work of every frequent flyer. The specific steps to do this are given in detail in part two of this book. In the meantime the ideas behind this approach are more useful here. Let's go ahead and cement our understanding of what we are trying to do and why. To start with, when it comes to man against the environment the environment always wins. Fighting this fact is useless so finding a workaround is the next best thing. Finding the answer is not that hard as a precedent has already been set. In any environment man has thrived in he adapted to the environment or brought his own environment with him. Living in any extreme environment is a prime example of this. Eskimos and hermits are some of the examples that spring to mind. They live in harsh environments and manage to overcome them by being able to adapt. Building vitality is our master key to making that adaptation work when we fly.

Questions

- How do you currently manage the three constants?

- What will you change if you change anything at all?

- Do you have suggestions of what a right type of solution might look like? Jot them down and compare with part two of this book.

CHAPTER 6

Why Flying Has Changed and So Must You

Globalization

Flying has been profoundly affected by the growing globalization of the world economies, so please forgive me if I come across as scholarly in attempting to explain its impact on flying. It is important to have this understanding in order to measure impact and the direction commercial aviation is heading. It is only with this knowledge that we can see how important it is to play for the long term.

Globalization has been described as the process of making the world economies more integrated or more interdependent; with that definition successive waves of globalization started in the 1870s. The second wave started in the post-war world of 1945. The most recent wave, like all the ones before it, led to an increase in the wealth of nations, which in flying terms translates to more people flying, be it for business or pleasure.

Industries and companies can seek markets across borders due to globalization and often do; it is summed up by the phrase "the world is your oyster" or the more appropriate "the world is your marketplace." The global marketplace expands on this phrase alone as more money and resources (including more travel by air) go into exploring the potential of these marketplaces.

Anything from having eyes and ears on the ground to nominating local representatives to carry out business on a company's behalf requires some form of movement of people across the globe. The research and development (R&D) industries undertake in order to grow may require the movement of goods and services across borders, again made possible by flying goods and people all around the world.

To date globalization has supported an upward growth trend of the gross domestic product (GDP) of nations around the world. This has sustained and fueled the commercial aviation enterprise for the best part of its history. It continues to play a driving role in the increased numbers of people flying as is demonstrated by the growing powerhouse economies of China, India and the emerging markets.

U.S. President George W. Bush

After curtly telling a reporter that jet lag was to blame for being "off his game," George W. Bush tried to leave a November 2005 press conference in China through a locked set of doors.

Source: http://content.time.com/time/specials/packages/article/0,28804, 1872183_1872185_1872181,00.html

This increase in GDP means as nations have more to buy and sell to each other the increase in wealth of these nations trickles into all parts of the society and pulls more people out of relative poverty. Economies get bigger and trade more; the industries in these countries do the same too. The people involved in these industries and who work for these companies also benefit and thus is born a middle class ready to prime the pump of business and leisure travel.

The increased rate of globalization is historically an indicator of increased global travel demand. A discussion paper titled "The Future for Interurban Passenger Transport - Bringing Citizens Closer Together" presented to the International Transport Research Symposium of 2009 [1] confirms this much. Globalization itself is being driven by rapid adoption, use and spread of information and technology. Globalization makes the world a more competitive place and technology is seen as one tool that can give companies an advantage over the competition. As a result, innovation and technological turnover are increasing rapidly as a means to stay ahead of the pack, and this in turn is fueling more globalization.

The fact that globalization is fueling GDP growth rates the world over is not set to change any time soon. Even with the global financial crisis of 2008, aviation still had a relatively positive outlook. This was because marketplaces like India and China, with their emerging middle class, were able to pick up the slack and keep the ball rolling. As long as their GDP figures and the figures of the other emerging market nations coming up behind them create more disposable income, airline travel figures will continue to be strong even if they do dip or remain flat for some periods.

The strong airline travel figures create a desirable problem for airlines. How do they satisfy the demand created with limited resources? This leads to the question: what does globalization growth mean in terms of impact on aviation? This is the second factor we are set to consider as we look at how flying has changed.

The Industry's Demands of Flying

As the world has globalized it has also mobilized. Through time the most obvious way increased demand has affected the airline operators has been the expansion of their operating schedules. According to the economic winds at specific times, airlines have increased or decreased their flying schedules in a number of ways. On the whole this has been trending upward even if there have been blips along the way. The measures to do this include increasing frequency or capacity. For example, creating a larger reach through an airline growing its own network of routes and markets or piggybacking on the networks of its code-sharing partners.

Since the beginning of the commercial aviation industry, innovation and technology have continued to push the boundaries in terms of achieving more efficiency. Initially the push was exclusively in the area of infrastructure, whether it is in the building of airports or the planes themselves. We went from the propeller engine and flying boats to the jet engine and the more efficient jet engine. We have also gone from the manual flight controls to fly-by-wire technology. Through trial, error and loss of life, the airline industry has implemented rules, regulations and safeguards to make the flying journey safer and without incident. The thrust of that efficiency drive also extends to the labor employed to run the airlines, which also includes flying crews.

Airlines have come to the realization that a plane on the ground is a plane losing money. Turning planes around as quickly as possible is the goal. As it takes crews to fly the planes, crew idle on the ground also means potential loss for airlines. As a combined result of the economics of demand and efficiency, planes and crew spending weeks on end at destinations is largely a thing of the past.

Early on in my flying career I had heard of 21-day Australia trips with crews spending weeks at a time in one location. In 17 years of flying I am yet to spend seven days at any one location even when there has been a technical problem with the plane causing it to be grounded. The longest trip on the network (for the airline I work for) at the moment is a nine-day Australia trip made up of two nights in Bangkok or Singapore on the way to Sydney, one night in Sydney, turning around, two nights in Bangkok or Singapore on the way back and arriving in London on day nine – how times have changed!

The efficient use of resources is welcome and necessary in any business that wishes to remain profitable and in business. The challenge in this situation is for an industry as complex as the airline industry to manage to keep up the desired productivity levels it requires to be successful when it has:

- A workforce that travels the world constantly

- A workforce that is ageing quickly with the passage of time

- A workforce habitually exposed to much uncertainty in the course of carrying out its duties (for uncertainty read stress)

More to the point, how does an airline do this with a workforce that has to contend with jet lag as an occupational hazard? This is a question the airlines and the industry are failing to answer in my opinion, but before we get to that there is one more thing the industry demands of flying that has come into sharper focus with the advent of the world becoming smaller through globalization.

Information and communication are the major drivers that make the world smaller through their ability to impact events faster than they could do before. The time lag that once existed between an event and its effect has shortened so dramatically that they have the power to upset and change events around the globe at a moment's notice. This is a headache frequent flyers and airlines have to deal with on an ongoing basis.

Responding to these events takes resources of all kinds including human resources; as the saying goes, it's not the absence of problems that keeps the customer coming back but how one handles the problems. A great example I heard recently was from the BBC Radio 4 program *The Bottom Line* with Evan Davis [2] focusing on the travel industry. Carolyn McCall of EasyJet explained that the Icelandic ash cloud debacle that disrupted northern European flight paths cost EasyJet £58 million to get their passengers back home even though it was no fault of EasyJet's. In Carolyn's own words "it was the right thing to do." The greatest resource in uncertain times like this can often be the human element and creativity brought to the table to find solutions.

The constant changing events in the geopolitical world we now live in holds uncertainty for all flyers and an even greater cry for a sense of security. The carefree certainty that used to exist pre 9/11 has evaporated and flyers are constantly reminded of this fact every time they pass through rigorous pat-downs at airport security.

U.S. President Barack Obama

A 2010 presidential health report for President Obama suggests a prescription drug was given to help the president survive the perils of jet lag while on international diplomatic duty.

Source: The Presidential Approach to Jet Lag http://maphappy.org/2014/04/presidential-approach-jet-lag/

For travelers in certain circumstances, when the unexpected happens the only source of security is the knowledge that they can at least get back home. At times like this, flying crews are front and center in being some kind of reassurance to travelers in a strange land or amidst the uncertainty. This reassuring role, whether overt or covert in the familiar friendliness of the cabin crew, the welcoming PA message of the captain or the sight of the familiar tailfin, is all brought into sharper focus against the uncertainty faced in the world out there. As such, obstacles to how these people perform or don't perform matter. The aviation industry has to get on board and actively participate in making sure the creativity and prescience of their people matters in the key clutch moments like these.

The Changed Job Description of Flying in the 21st Century

I may have already busted the myth that flying as crew is as glamorous as it was once thought to be but it is important to make this distinction. The job flying crew actually do is not the job most of the population see in their mind's eye when they think of crew. It is not all swanky hotels, cocktail bars, endless time in the world's best locations and drunken reveries. That is not to say there are not benefits to doing the job but it now takes so much more out of crew to do the job than before.

The problem is that crew themselves, the airlines they work for and a majority of the public still have the outdated view of the job. The specific problem for crew is that quite a few of them do live the job like they were back in the good old days! This is a dangerous issue for the crew as it can cost them their livelihood and health if they are not careful. It is not particularly good for the airlines as they start hemorrhaging crew and cannot maintain the balance of experience and youth the flying image demands.

But this isn't a sob story. I'm not saying that crew have it particularly bad or are worse off than any other profession, but I am saying the stresses of the job have become more intensified over time and no one is addressing them properly. As the industry has grown the workload has changed and where you could once be assured of enough time off wherever you went to recuperate, you now leave after minimum rest.

The accumulation of trips where rest is down to the minimum (which is all trips for an efficiently run airline) coupled with the stress we all face in life leaves no room for endless round the world parties. Flying crew experience burnout on a similar scale to multinational corporate traveling executives. A combination of factors makes this a reality crew face every day: constant body clock shifts, maximized flying schedules, living in the 21st century and the rise of stress and deficient autoimmunity.

In following the occupational health medical literature it is quite clear that flying crew are a category of shift workers and as a result they are prone to the same challenges. Health challenges for shift workers stem mainly from the disorder of melatonin patterns. (This is also a trait among non-crew frequent flyers.) They include problems with hormones generally, and specifically sleep, certain types of cancers and stress. Google *The Journal of Occupational and Environmental Health* and *melatonin* for examples of how disruptive shift work can be.

Flying crew find themselves in this position from a combination of latitudinal travel, which triggers melatonin release suppression, and from working through the night. Once upon a time, with youth on their side, crew could ride out the challenges of these factors with ample amounts of natural growth hormone.

As crew age and the growth hormone secretions naturally decline, their ability to cope recedes and the negative effects are felt more keenly. This has always been the case as human biochemistry is predictable and does not change so willingly but we have only started to see the effects because we are only starting to see a lifetime of flying as we see professional flyers of 20, 30 and 40 years come out the other end. As well as the physical stresses of the job you also have the mental and emotional stress of frequent flying. As an infrequent flyer, you may ask how stressful can handing out chicken or beef be. But the job entails more than meets the eye.

All types of flying crew spend about half the year in the air, which means you have to squeeze everything else everyone else does into half the time. This by itself can be stressful and if you factor in other people's demands on your time, social commitments, mandatory functions and the requirements of healthy home relationships it soon adds up. Keeping a lid on it all is an art form and is a lesson in never-ending gap analysis. When you close the gap in one area another gap has opened somewhere else and so on ad infinitum.

Going away on an average of once a week means you constantly have to check back into relationships. When most flying crew started flying they were probably young and single. Stability and mature relationships were probably not high on the agenda but as crew progress in the job, tastes, preferences and priorities change. These changes often bring about stresses and tensions within relationships if not tended carefully, and being away so often doesn't help. Anyone who doesn't fly for a living will find it hard to understand and it is often the case that when a couple consists of a flyer and a non-flyer the relationship suffers for this very reason.

It's my experience of crew that half of them can't wait to get away from home to have a break from the stresses of home and the other half are stressed because they can't wait to get back to their home life. As you can imagine, working in the airline industry with its uncertainty and complexity will give these people challenges to their relationships at some point in their flying career.

Crew are usually able to hide the details of their personal life quite well but every now and then the mask slips. When it slips spectacularly you get stories like the JetBlue captain ranting about terrorists and Al-Qaeda or the JetBlue flight attendant who screamed at passengers and pulled an emergency chute and left, or the American Airlines flight attendant who lost it, screaming and claiming not to be responsible for plane crashes over the PA system. For the most part, crew keep the mental and emotional stresses of the job in check on the plane and might take it out in the bar after the flight. For some this is an ideal way to work through the stress (if they don't abuse alcohol). In some cases when that is not an option the stress can build up to barely manageable levels.

One of the first tools taught in training school is how to manage the varying degrees of stress the job may present; some crew are able to do this better than others. When it builds up like in the examples above and becomes habitual, crew tend to look for outlets in all manner of things: outrageous antics, drunken loud room parties and drugs are known to be a few. I've heard of flight crew flying the plane naked and cabin crew landing in from Africa snorting Class A drugs under blankets in the rear galley. All in all they are signs of needing to get release from whatever stressful burden they have.

Some airlines are more aware of the mental and emotional stresses the job poses and support their crews with remedial tools. I know of a Spanish airline that used to give their incoming crew a psychological evaluation as part of their recruitment process. One U.K. airline provides a counseling service for its crew. The fact that these services exist is a sign of the times and recognition that flying crew need extra support as the job has changed.

To really understand what all the fuss is about you have to get that variety and change is a big part of crew life and, like all human beings, we want a level of stability we can rely on at some level. When that certainty is not available from whatever source we usually get it from, stress ensues. A good metaphor to explain this is flying itself: as crew spend a lot of their time in the clouds, some source of grounding is an important element of their lives.

I mentioned above that some crew like to live in the good old days of flying. This is a changing picture as change is being forced upon them by events and new circumstances. Some of the relics of that old mindset relate specifically to how they look after themselves. Once upon a time, crew would party like there was no tomorrow safe in the knowledge that they had a few days to recover before making the journey back. Crew also used to view exercise as optional. They thought they could eat whatever they liked without it affecting their weight while on the job. They viewed flying as a stopgap before you went off and got a "proper" job or got married.

Nowadays crew are at least aware that common sense practice is to do some kind of exercise, eat a healthy diet to complement their lifestyle and not burn the candle at both ends. These are further signs the job has changed. Crew who ignore this most basic common sense advice store up problems for themselves as their careers progress. Sickness and absenteeism figures in airlines are beginning to show this much.

Health Status and Autoimmune Deficiency

The first prerequisite of flying crew is health. Most airlines will test this in some shape or form during the recruitment process. While some airlines leave the issue of health testing at that, health on a global scale is changing for everyone. You may have heard the refrain already: rising obesity, reduced fertility, increased disability, increased projected cancer rates, reduced immunity, and the list goes on. What is alarming some observers is the global population's seemingly reduced ability to fight back. We are witnessing a pandemic of autoimmune deficiency.

A report from the American Autoimmune Related Disease Association (AARDA) confirms what many others had spoken about and what doctors worldwide were experiencing in their practices on a daily basis. The report "A Briefing Report on Autoimmune Diseases and AARDA: Past Present and Future" [3] highlights two important facts all airlines should take note of. The first is that autoimmune deficiency is more prevalent among women than men. Any employer with a large female workforce should take note. The second point made was that causes of autoimmune disease relate to heredity, epigenetics and environmental factors. While airlines can do nothing about the first two factors, environmental triggers may be something they can address within the workplace. Three types of cancer identified as being prevalent among crew show a workplace environment bias, i.e. they are occupationally related.

How does this information impact airlines and flying crew specifically? Airlines have had a history of recruiting the young and healthy because they know the job is grueling.

They figure if they get them young and healthy they can get the best out of them while they are still young enough to take the punishment frequent flying metes out! Guess what? The young are not so healthy anymore and unless they buck the trend by being brought up on an island untouched by globalization and modern living they will never be again!

This trend of lowered autoimmunity is so far-reaching that experts and observers are saying that 80% of all illnesses have an autoimmune deficiency aspect to them. In effect this means that recruitment drives by airlines will yield a comparatively more expensive workforce as time goes by. More sickness at airlines means less productivity and less efficiency.

In case you are in any doubt, immunity and autoimmunity are crucially important aspects of health for flying crew. I'd go as far as to say travel requires immunity. Crew fly to far corners of the globe weekly and come into contact with all types of environments with different peculiarities, some of which are not necessarily friendly to non-natives.

Crews carry millions of passengers in a metal tube in a low oxygen environment, which is conducive to spreading germs, bacteria and viruses. They do all this while compromising their health with nights out of bed, a physically demanding job, occupationally triggered hormone imbalances and whatever other personal stresses they may be under.

In many ways immunity parallels another important factor in flying: the environment. Flying from A to B in a metal tube requires a stable environment. Maintaining immunity gives rise to a stable internal environment in which we function. Autoimmunity is a step beyond that as it allows us to take aspects of our health for granted without us having to focus our attention on them. Just as immunity and autoimmunity protect us from invaders of all kinds, the aircraft environment protects us when traveling. I raise this point now because it is an idea we will revisit again when we get to look at healthy jet lag solutions. It is important to get your head around seeing your immunity as an extension of your protective environment.

I said it before and I say it again here, technology is both sinner and saint in our approach to flying better. In this instance we are going to concentrate on the undesirable elements of technology that contribute to reduced autoimmunity. Just as technology is taking us forward to greater standards of living, it is impacting the lives of everyone and everything on the planet. An example of the negative impact specific to autoimmunity is in the broadened use of radio frequency (RF) waves in the confines of the aircraft cabin.

Through the use of radio waves man has harnessed the powers of the ether like never before. With it we have also introduced new words into our vocabulary such as electrosmog and electrosensitivity. Our airwaves are literally riddled with these waves that make up our environment. The curious thing about environments is that just as we influence them they influence us.

The mass of electromagnetic signals we use to navigate our worlds also has a physical impact on our bodies. While these signals have been harnessed to run our technologies, the impact they have on our bodies is damaging. This is especially so when it comes down to the ionizing and non-ionizing radiation content they pass on to the user as a by-product of use.

I have best heard the barrage of electronic signals we are bombarded with explained like this. Imagine if you could hear the wave signature of that Wi-Fi signal from your base station as it travels through the air to you. It might sound something like duh-duh-duh-duh with a beat every three seconds. Now imagine the wireless signal from a mobile phone, it might have a beat of a signal every millisecond. These signals are constantly bombarding our physiology on a daily basis; as they do so they cause low-level chronic stress.

The chronic stress these technologies give us is overloading our immunity in ways that are just beginning to be understood. Even if you refuse to participate in the gadget-filled way of living in the 21st century, your neighbor's router and mobile signals can travel through the walls of the building and affect you. There is literally no place to hide.

Just as we had the curious cases of increased occurrences of leukemia near powerful electricity pylons, changes in our environment caused by this use of radio frequency waves have been tracked and shown to cause damage to the environment we live in at large. I quote the research done by the multi-disciplined BioInitiative Working Group whose paper "The BioInitiative Report" made some very revealing observations about our use of radio waves. The extremely low frequencies (ELFs) are causing particular damage to our habitat. A bit closer to home, literally, there are people who are now being diagnosed with electrosensitivity health challenges.

These people are acutely sensitive to ionizing and non-ionizing radiation from all gadgets and can only use some of these tools for short periods of time without becoming stressed or it becoming painful. In Sweden this illness is now so recognized that the government has set aside grants for people suffering from this illness to build protective housing [4].

If it is not bad enough that our homes are minefields of electromagnetic activity, the workplace is even worse. Insulation and closed system air conditioning (not unlike plane air conditioning) compound the problem while computers, faxes and digital gadgets generate emissions and radiation. At home at least you could escape to the outdoors and reconnect with nature to get some kind of respite. In office blocks people work long hours in the artificially created environments, often without breaks, all the while being bombarded with ionizing and non-ionizing radiation. So people go from home to work and back home all the while under the influence of low-level chronic stress caused by our relationship with technology.

In the case of flying crew it is from home to the plane and back home. The plane, which is a unique environment already under the influence of cosmic radiation and the other listed influences, is under threat of further destruction with the introduction of Wi-Fi on planes.

While it may be popular with the traveling public who want to connect to the office or watch a movie, it spells disaster as a working environment. On a plane radiation from Wi-Fi is more dangerous than it can be on the ground. On the ground the denser oxygen-rich atmosphere we live in naturally protects the Earth. At altitude the barometric pressure is thinner, which means there is less oxygen in the air. Less oxygen means less protection. To make matters worse, if you are working in this kind of environment week in week out it becomes a habitual danger.

Technology is virtually killing us. Mobile and Wireless although convenient and revolutionary are causing an attachment to gadgets that is unhealthy. A recent infographic by the company PC Housing called "Mobile Dependence: A Growing Trend in Business Travel" [5] crunches the data to show how addicted business travelers really are. While we may not all be business travelers, looking at the infographic reveals habits around technology we can all relate to, so no one is off the hook.

This addiction to technology is the forerunner of another trend worth highlighting to everyone who wants to deal naturally with jet lag and healthy flying. It is the habit of being connected 24/7. The always on, always available habit we are cultivating is ramping stress up through the roof and doesn't allow down time to switch off. A notable observation to make is that the deeper involvement we have with technology, the more we have moved away from our immemorial connection with our natural habitat.

Our connection to Earth is a source of infinite rejuvenation potential. As generations have moved off the land and sought the bright lights and big cities of the Industrial Age, that lost connection which benefited us well in the past is in retreat.

Not to put too fine a point on it, the clue is in the language used to describe some of the symptoms of jet lag and flying. People say they feel spaced out after long flights and need to get "grounded." As a frequent flyer looking for a natural preventative cure for jet lag, getting grounded is a habit all flyers should cultivate. Research shows that the Earth's surface is teeming with an inexhaustible supply of electrons, which are shown to be the ultimate supply of antioxidants for the human body. Jump to "Protection" in part two of this book if you can't wait.

Our dependency on technology feeds directly into overwhelming our physiology and affects health. This is a major way technology feeds into the autoimmune deficiency pandemic mentioned earlier. As technology isn't planning to pack up and go home or stop affecting our lives, urgent steps need to be taken by all flyers who value their health. That is not to say I advocate abandoning technology altogether. What we must do is make it safe and this starts when we start to become aware of the price we pay for our ignorance.

While most of the examples I have used in this chapter relate to flying crew – pilots and cabin crew – I am sure other types of frequent flyers can relate to the way flying has changed and continues to change over the years. The point I am trying to get across to all types of flyers is that this change requires us to change in response if we are to remain relevant to the businesses we serve, the businesses we run and the meaningful relationships and lives we lead. It is better to be in a position to see the change coming and have the ability to act and stay competitive rather than be in reaction all the time and have limited or no control. You could pretty much substitute any kind of frequent or business traveler for crew in the scenarios above; they all face these same challenges.

Questions

- How much tech gear do you travel with? Are you aware of how addictive it is and how it can interfere with melatonin release?

- As a flyer do you measure your health status regularly?

- Do you have any preventative measures in place to replace what globetrotting takes out of you?

CHAPTER 7

Challenges Unique to Frequent Flyers

As a frequent flyer do you recognize that the deck is stacked, and it is not in your favor? Part of understanding the type of world frequent flyers inhabit leads us to a set of challenges all frequent flyers face. Time and again, especially when there are health challenges to be handled, I hear of flyers who go to their primary healthcare practitioners for help and advice. The well-intentioned practitioner sees the flyer as no different from any other patient who walks into their surgery or office, and treats them as such. The results have tended to be less than satisfactory. Good intentions on the part of the physician are admirable, but to really help flyers an understanding of some of the unique challenges they face is helpful to both physician and flyer alike.

Such an understanding will help any type of physician put their skills and expertise to best use for the flyer and it will help the flyer come to terms with what they put their body through when flying. Hopefully it will also help them come to the realization that they must take remedial steps to maintain their health over and above the norms considered by non-flyers. Self-knowledge is especially powerful to the flyer, as the stresses of travel will tend to manifest through our constitutional weaknesses. While not exhaustive these are some of the challenges frequent flyers face as a group.

The Hormonal Seesaw

Latitudinal travel is the most influential on the human body because depending on which direction you go you will encounter longer days or shorter nights and thus alter the habitual pattern of the body clock. The amount of light perceived by the eyes is the cue which helps regulate the ongoing hormonal cascade that keeps the body functioning as it should.

This cue is known in chronobiology as a Zeitgeber. While there are other Zeitgebers and rhythms that help regulate functions across the body, science is confirming that in some way they all take their cues from the amount of light perceived in the eye. The pathway is thought to involve the suprachiasmatic nuclei (SNC) in the head and the melatonin found in this part of the body, which together form part of the body clock.

For frequent flyers (defined as flying once a week minimum) the constant need to adjust to the different amounts of daylight based on where in the world you go is a stressful challenge to the physiology. One of the scientific clues to this is the research already referred to, carried out by the University of Durham, which looked at the amount of cortisol found in stewardesses' saliva on long- and short-haul routes. Just to recap, the researchers found cortisol levels among the long-haul stewardesses to be elevated more than the samples taken from the short-haul stewardesses. It concluded that long-haul flying predisposed the stewardesses to more stress than short-haul flying. While the results only looked specifically at cortisol, I would suggest it is safe to draw the conclusion that other hormones would be challenged or out of sync based on the fact that the hormonal system works in concert via a biofeedback loop.

U.S. President George H.W. Bush

In 1992 President George H.W. Bush vomits on himself and over his host, the Japanese Prime Minister Miyazawa, at a state dinner. Marlin Fitzwater, the president's spokesperson, later put it down to gastroenteritis. Given Bush's extensive 12-day, 26,000-mile itinerary, it is quite possible that his condition was brought on by jet lag.

Source: Dan Caldwell & William Hocking, "Jet Lag: A Neglected Problem of Modern Diplomacy?" *The Hague Journal of Diplomacy* 9.3 (2014): 281-295

If you look at the health histories of flying crews as a group, many of them also tend to have issues around hormone-related themes such as weight gain (insulin), metabolism (thyroid), and fertility (male and female sex hormones). The intelligence of the human body does its best to handle the disruption to its normal flow of rhythms mediated by the hormonal system but it can only do its best in the face of the continued disruption and so we have the ongoing hormonal seesaw to contend with as frequent flyers.

Routines and Habits

Keeping up routines and habits is one of the best things frequent flyers can do in the face of a world where they are constantly landing into different time zones and making the required adjustments. In a sense, routines and habits are a way to give back the regularity and timing lost in the constant change the lifestyle forces upon flyers. As odd as it might sound, habits and routines really do kick your body into a groove. When you connect with the familiar, your body responds too, it knows and anticipates what is next.

Having some routines that are set in stone no matter where you are in the world is a good way to get around any lethargy you may have and a way of telling your body what time it is for you. You may agree or disagree with this depending on how much you accept the notion that clock time is an artificial construct of man. Its power lies in the fact that we have wielded ourselves to its patterns but we are free to set new ones as we please, provided we do it with consistency and enough practice.

It doesn't matter if you are a lark or an owl in my opinion, what matters is that you have routines in place wherever you go to give you back your sense of time. Being able to establish this sense of time is important; many a time in my early years of flying I remember being asked what day of the week it was and not being able to respond correctly. For flyers it is easy to lose track of time, routines can help you create time stamps.

While we are on the subject of time I find it helpful to use an expanded understanding of what time is. I think of time as clock time and body time, external time and internal time respectively. External time is what we are taught to set our schedules and the ebb and flow of our lives to, it is linear. Internal time is the time governed by what occurs in the body. To my mind, proof of this exists in the fact that the biochemistry of the body has its own sequences it follows, which have been found to be more or less independent of linear time.

This means as long as you can influence the body's biochemistry you can in effect influence its perception of time. Tell your body what time it is. You do this already when you travel so you might as well do it consciously and use it to your best advantage. This is based on the knowledge that your biochemistry in the morning is quite different from your biochemistry in the evening. The fact that there is a sequence suggests there is an element of timing involved; manipulating that timing or making it flexible makes all the difference.

The challenge lies in having these routines and sticking to them no matter what while on the road. In terms of health, flyers would do well to set up routines and habits around exercise and wellness. Habits around getting up and going to bed, meal times and nap times are equally important as they tend to slip when the unexpected shows up in the itinerary. It is impossible to get it right 100% of the time but the idea is to have enough discipline through the practice of the routines to be able to get back in the groove when you are knocked off course. If done properly, tools like these help build drive and that invaluable well of vitality needed for the road.

Grounding

The saying goes that if God meant us to fly he would have given us wings. Further evidence that he meant us to have our two feet firmly planted on the ground is that we have geomagnetic forces emanating from the Earth's core which are supportive to our health. As noted in chapter 3 this force is an inexhaustible source of electrons, which are the ultimate antioxidants of the body. Connecting with this unlimited supply of antioxidants is rejuvenating and best of all it is free.

Frequent flyers on the other hand spend a lot of their time in the air away from the influence of the Earth's lower atmosphere and cut off from this aforementioned rejuvenating source. For the most part, all inhabitants who walk on the Earth with rubber-soled shoes also cut themselves off from this source of free energy, but they don't suffer as much because they don't fly as much. Because frequent flyers are flying every week they are further disconnected from this nourishing source of energy in other ways too. They fly in a metal tube across the Earth's magnetic fields getting further out of sync, literally turning day into night and vice versa. They arrive frazzled and disoriented and leave in that same state of being.

U.S. Secretary of State John Kerry

Secretary of State John Kerry: "I can't say my past experiments with jet lag remedies have been very scientific. When I'm flying, I usually take an Ambien and listen to one of my own speeches on my iPod. I'm out in seconds."

Source: The Presidential Approach to Jet Lag http://maphappy.org/2014/04/presidential-approach-jet-lag/

When the flyers arrive home they are truly whacked, out of sorts and have many symptoms that contribute to jet lag. One of the simplest things they could do is go outside and connect with the Earth barefoot for 45 minutes to feel the healing energy of the Earth drain all the static and cancel out the positive ions they accumulated during the journey. It has been noted under clinical conditions that the simple act of grounding yourself sets physiological markers like blood pressure and heart beat heading back to healthy norms.

Grounding the body evens out the balance of electrical energy in the body, that is basically how grounding works. As we go about our day-to-day lives we naturally create lots of toxins internally and from the environment around us. These interactions create positively charged by-products that must be neutralized. Grounding is the great neutralizer. Simply put, grounding restores a healthful charge to the body.

Flying with all its stress, fatigue and disorientation upsets this healthy charge. Rebalancing this charge is a shortcut to beating jet lag at the cellular level and is a tool every flyer would do well to use on a regular basis. The result of not discharging this positive charge is a more acid environment which the body has to use precious resources, usually in short supply, to neutralize.

An over acid environment is not a good starting point from which to try and manifest balanced health. Not only does acidity make it an uphill struggle for any healthcare practitioner assisting in a wellness program but it is also a distinct disadvantage when the flyer steps onboard a plane, as the plane environment will only worsen the situation.

Energy Bankruptcy

Although it is partly related to sleep I am singling out energy as a unique challenge because a lack of energy undermines the ability to function properly in anything we may wish to accomplish. Energy bankruptcy among frequent flyers is rife and of epic proportions. Most deal with it on a day-to-day basis instead of taking a long-term view, and this is part of the problem. Those who don't deal with it at all often find themselves showing symptoms of adrenal fatigue. For the majority, the other symptom of energy bankruptcy is weight gain or yoyo weight gain and weight loss.

Erratic eating habits, poor choice of foods and the energy demands of flying all contribute to this problem. More often than not the easiest thing to do is to eat whatever is available. The problem is it is not always the best or healthiest choice.

Another point in this energy equation is when flyers do eventually have time off from flying they have to manage the affairs of their lives in half the time the non-flyers do. This in itself can be stressful if they are always playing catch-up. Sometimes it seems like frequent flyers are on a never-ending hamster wheel. They find it hard to make time to get the vital rest they need before they head out flying again. If they fail to address this problem the long-term danger is they exhaust themselves and again manifest adrenal fatigue. This can be brought about from over exertion and the use of stimulants, which tap into emergency energy supplies without the ability to make good the deficit.

Sleep Quality

While the media is full of reports of how we are all sleeping less, the frequent flyer's challenge is more specific: sleep quality. It is one thing to miss a good night's sleep while traveling (frequent flyers are notorious for not sleeping well on planes) but it is another to go to bed for a good eight hours and still wake up tired. Sleeping and being well rested are two different things. Sleep labs the world over are all turning out research that proves we are worse off from a lack of a good night's sleep. Productivity, cognition and memory are a few things known to be impaired as a result. Coupled with energy bankruptcy, the downward health spiral continues. In my experience, unless something is done about it the impact is felt mentally first with consequences for all other areas of life.

Part of the problem is that sleep is never taken seriously as a resource, and yes in the past I have been guilty of this too! It is easy to see it as a hindrance if you have a busy life and your to do list has a to do list! But sleep is a resource as science is now proving to us. We house clean our minds and do the deep filing we are unable to do during the waking hours. It is said that during sleep is the only time when nerve energy is replenished. We need this energy to get through the day.

The sooner we see sleep as a resource, the sooner we will cultivate better sleep habits. In the meantime though there are tools and technology available right now which help you get better quality sleep and also help you chart your way back to better sleeping practices. My guess is that because sleep is not valued as it should be these tools remain largely unknown or unused.

The only real solution to sleep challenges is to anticipate them and hard-wire the solutions into your lifestyle. If you do this habitually as a frequent flyer you can avoid most of the pitfalls. The solutions themselves may look different for each flyer depending on the kind of lifestyle they lead but there are basics that everyone can benefit from. Some of the stock advice doing the rounds is:

- Go to bed at the same time

- Sleep in a completely dark room

- Avoid noise or disturbances when sleeping

- Get up the same time every day

- Don't become excitable just before bed

- Don't eat a heavy meal before bed

All of these aren't particularly easy to comply with if you are always traveling so some modifications are in order. I think it is best to try to keep to the spirit of the advice. Personally I tend to go to bed as soon as I can when I land somewhere after my normal bedtime. I always sleep with the lights off and go so far as to turn any luminous bedside table clocks away from my line of sight or cover them up to make sure the room is dark.

I remember doing a particularly tiring flight into Nassau and collapsing into bed, only to awaken halfway through the night to the sound of noisy air conditioning. The following morning I went down to reception to request a room change. Looking out for disturbing white noise is always a good idea as a means to avoid interrupted sleep.

Getting up at the same time is really a nonstarter for frequent flyers; you have no control over the airline schedules so you may often find yourself getting up at odd times to catch flights and make it to the airport. The main gauge I use is how well rested I feel when I wake. Not getting too excitable before bed usually means not watching emotionally ridden TV programs or exercising just before bed; add doing anything that dramatically changes your biochemistry to that.

Not eating heavy meals goes without saying, as the physical discomfort will keep you awake if nothing else. The only addition of note I would add to this list particular to flyers is the habit of using gadgets in bed. There is growing evidence that it shuts off the release of melatonin thereby making it harder to fall asleep. As difficult as it may be, you have to turn the gadgets off. I like to read in the evening and turning off my iPad used to be a challenge; I've taken to reading on an Amazon Kindle which doesn't reflect light.

Australian Prime Minister Tony Abbott

Australian Prime Minister Tony Abbott renames Canada "Canadia" when making remarks about Canada's response to Russian/ Ukrainian affairs, put down to being jet lagged.

Source: http://news.nationalpost.com/news/canada/ welcome-to-canadia-tony-australian-prime-ministers- brief-verbal-slip-up-a-vowel-too-far-for-social-media

---

Going back to routines and habits, I do my best to make a consistent routine out of the inconsistency that is my flying lifestyle, and I advise you to do the same. If the same challenge keeps showing up and interrupting your sleep "routine" it means it hasn't been properly anticipated and you need to go back to the drawing board. On the other hand, sometimes circumstances are beyond your control and the only thing you can do is do whatever it takes to keep your sanity and wait for things to return to normal.

Adrenal Fatigue

I almost didn't include adrenal fatigue [1] because the title of this chapter is challenges unique to frequent flyers. Well you don't have to be a flyer to have adrenal fatigue, this type of fatigue is a characteristic that shows up quite often in the health picture of flyers. When it is chronic it can go unnoticed but when it becomes acute it can be very disruptive.

It is important to mention as adrenal problems can play a behind the scene role in flyer health challenges that are hormone related and because of what east-west flying does to hormonal balance. It is, however, a medical condition best dealt with by you and with the help of your primary healthcare practitioner.

Questions

- Do any of these themes sound familiar to you? Are you working with a healthcare professional who understands the role being a frequent flyer plays in your life?

- What kind of challenges do you have with sleep? Duration, quality, sleeping on planes, background noise? What solutions have you used to remedy the situation?

CHAPTER 8

The Outcomes of a Jetspert

What is a Jetspert?

A Jetspert is a **Jet Stress Expert** [1]. Someone versed in the art of frequent travel who makes the smoothest transition or adaptation to the time and environment they find themselves in without suffering the usual drawbacks of jet lag. In my 17 plus years of flying I have come across individuals who have mastered some aspects of the art of flying healthily but not others. Either through a lack of know-how or not being able to connect the many dots, they are unable to distinguish the differences that make the difference in results. This is a salute to them and their efforts to beat the healthy flying odds. They are the original Jetsperts even if they had crude tools or understood the process imprecisely.

A Jetspert is someone who lives the lifestyle of a frequent flyer and knows enough about the flying experience to be able to negate the negative impact of flying on their performance. They understand that being a healthy frequent flyer is a lifestyle choice. They live that way for the benefit of their health and productivity and as a person who has enough energy to live a fully balanced life when not flying. Becoming a Jetspert is about moving from conscious incompetence to unconscious competence on the subject of flying well.

Through this book, which explains the P.H.A.R.E. Well System of healthy flying and jet lag elimination, it is my intention to show you how to become a Jetspert in the sky. Traveling well is a skill useful to any flyer who travels with a purpose especially when it comes to excelling in business and performance.

Helpful Distinctions

My stated aim is to show you how to fly while banishing jet lag and building vitality at the same time. I want to show you how to do it healthily and in a way that makes it second nature to you anytime you travel. In order to do this it is necessary to highlight and emphasize a few things you might already know but may not have realized the significance of. A coach of mine once impressed upon me the idea that he who is able to make the most distinctions on a given topic or item has the most power to influence. So with that in mind it is important to make the following distinctions that will allow you to travel well and eventually become a Jetspert:

- The Vitality Component

- The Toolbox

- The Habit of Self-Reliance

- Cultivating the Long-Term View of Beating Jet Lag

The Vitality Component

In choosing tools to beat jet lag it is important to select tools that build your energy and your energy base as the cornerstone of your strategy. I'm sure you've heard me say this enough times now but the majority of "cures" miss this vital component. It is key for the obvious reason: globetrotting is exhausting and takes a lot out of the traveler. You need to be able to replace the lost energy and more because you know you are going back on the road the next week. If you don't replace this energy you end up in a deficit.

The thing is we don't just want to play catch-up, we want to be ahead of the game. We want to have energy in abundance for all the other things we want to do, be and have in life. You need vitality to do this; if you are just replacing lost energy without building a surplus, globetrotting will take it out of you and then some!

One of the shorthand ideas of what this global travel thing is all about to me is this thing called Presence. I touched on it in the "Why the P.H.A.R.E. Well System is An Idea Whose Time Has Come for Frequent Flyers" chapter. When you travel are you really as present as you can be? In other words, do you show up fully as the best you can be? If not, why turn up at all? Can you say you are fully effective when you are not fully present? It doesn't matter about the circumstance, you need to be fully present before you can become fully engaged in whatever you are doing. If you do not consciously work at building vitality into your lifestyle as a frequent flyer, you can't possibly turn up and be fully present to achieve any worthwhile outcome. You just won't have the energy you need when you need it.

To make things worse, in this overstressed, fast-paced life you don't easily come across time outside of flying to build or acquire vitality. These are all home truths to any frequent flyer but what might not be so obvious is that the current ways people use to build energy are bankrupting them and taking them deeper into energy debt. They constantly borrow from their reserves of energy to help them get through the day without the realization that they need to pay it back. Instead of being able to pay it back they find themselves exhausted and deteriorating into adrenal fatigue and health issues.

A small percentage of frequent flyers know it's a good idea to prioritize working out regularly but are they working out and having enough time to fully recuperate, rest and rejuvenate? It can be hard to get that balance while on the road with lots going on around you. Building vitality is an active and passive activity. In the West we tend to focus too much on the active part of building vitality, to our detriment. The get up and go conqueror spirit compels us to go out there and do something to make it all happen; that's great but we also need the time to grow passively. We need that balance whether it's in the arena of physical fitness or any other energy we use.

The current crop of jet lag solutions don't address the vitality issue from this perspective with any seriousness. They think they do but they don't. The ones that try to address the energy question all take the same tack. They approach the problem from the perspective of stimulation. Their thinking is that as long as they can stimulate the body to produce energy, the problem is handled. The flip side is that once stimulation wears off you are further in deficit. What goes up must come down after all. If this is done repeatedly without some form of respite there comes a time when exhaustion and breakdowns are inevitable. All the more reason to make a conscious choice about how you choose to manage your energy and make building vitality one of your core distinctions.

The Toolbox

You might be a frequent flyer who clocks up the hours via point-to-point travel or a flyer who does an around the world trip and doesn't go to the same place twice. On the other hand, you might be somewhere in the middle. Whatever the case, and wherever go, you will want to have a variety of tools to help you adapt to different circumstances each time. As a Jetspert you will build yourself a toolbox of essentials that give you an edge and allow you to go anywhere and adapt as you wish.

Your toolbox will be based on your needs and requirements but it will be rooted in the same principles that apply to everyone who wishes to fly healthily. The more you understand the principles of healthy flying, the more you get to know what you need when and you build the toolbox with strategies and protocols that allow you to stay as flexible as needed.

It is worth pointing out here too that most ideas of what constitutes a tool tend to stick to pretty conventional or generic items. There is a growing list of tools from other disciplines and areas of life that are as useful to road warriors as they are to their native fields. Stepping outside the box and making use of these tools is something you will be able to do as a Jetspert – again, once you have grasped the principles of healthy flying this program is based upon.

The Habit of Self-Reliance

It goes without saying that when you are in a foreign country for the most part you are reliant on yourself. We certainly take that responsibility when it comes to our possessions. When it comes to getting what we need to make sure we have a healthy trip we can sometimes leave it to chance and depend on others or the hotel we are staying at. If enough people have passed through that journey and asked the same questions you are asking, you will probably be in luck and find the solution you seek. If on the other hand no one has, you are stuck with whatever you can find, which can be hit or miss.

As well as doing your prep before you leave, it is important to have an idea of what you want your healthy flying trip to look like and plan accordingly. I mean everything – all the way from what you can take through security to where you can get decent food, facilities, clean water, workout gear, where the nearest park is, everything. It is good to be able to have spontaneity when you travel too but don't let that stop you from meeting your prime objective to travel well.

Cultivating the Long-Term View of Beating Jet Lag

The law of instrument says if all you have is a hammer everything tends to look like a nail. Conversely, if you have made up your mind that overcoming jet lag is only a concern to you on a trip-by-trip basis it is unlikely you will look for tools that serve you beyond this purpose. The peddlers of current jet lag cures continually look at the challenges of jet lag in this manner. They bombard the marketing channels with this message so much that it seems this is the prevailing thought about jet lag. The problem is it is wrong and it stops any other view of the challenge taking root. If you have traveled much you will know from experience that these cures fall short, so what is the alternative? I would suggest taking the opposite view, a long-term view of the challenge of jet lag and frequent flying.

Cultivating the long-term view helps you align competing aspects of your life as a frequent flyer: your health, your use of time, productivity, your use of technology and nutrition and supplementation to name a few. When you begin to think of these items as having a meaning and an impact that affects your life in new ways, they increase in priority and become easier to incorporate into your life because you understand the payoff like never before. It is for this very reason that the frequent flyer's solution to jet lag that is healthy is a lifestyle solution rather than a trip-by-trip punt.

Questions

- Do you know any Jetsperts?

- What do they do particularly well?

- What could you mirror?

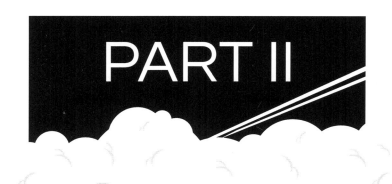

PART II

How to Fly Better Right Now the P.H.A.R.E. Well Way

Protect yourself from the damaging flying environment

Hydrate – stay hydrated throughout your travels and beyond

Acclimatize deftly at home and while on the road

Rhythms – master them and your body clock to stay in control

Environments – make the distinctions and master the environments that influence your health and flying

Wellness – make it a part of your lifestyle for benefits while flying and beyond

The P.H.A.R.E. Well System of Jet Lag Elimination and Prevention is a hybrid nutrition and fitness methodology. To benefit from this system all you the flyer has to do is follow the steps at your own pace. As you become more familiar with the steps you will begin to build greater resilience and vitality.

The Promise of the P.H.A.R.E. Well System of Jet Lag Elimination and Prevention:

1. Learn and master the principles and steps of this system and you will be fully present and engaged in whatever you do, wherever you go, no matter how often you travel to do it.

2. You will build a surplus of vitality that carries over to other areas of your life for you to do with as you please. You will beat jet lag and therefore jet stress long term.

3. You will have better tools to handle any underlying health challenges your frequent flying lifestyle exacerbates or highlights.

PROTECTION

This is where we take off. You have had the overview. This is the nuts and bolts view of the system. We delve into the specifics of each of the six steps first laid out in chapter 4. While there are specific principles you must stick to, viewing the P.H.A.R.E. Well System as a flexible tool is the best way to use it. Learn it and adapt it to your circumstances and needs.

Diet plays a central role in every single step at various stages of the solution's journey. There might be more detail than you are familiar with and you might see some repeating themes. This is intentional and serves to drive the point home. As a naturopathic nutritional therapist, nutritional therapy will always be the primary tool I use to explain solution options. While there may be other ways of getting the same results, I will most likely choose those related to nutrition, as it is what I notice first.

Always Stay Protected When You Fly

The requirement is that you see the aircraft cabin as an alien and compromised environment. As you cannot change it, protecting yourself from its compromising effects is the only way forward since you will be spending a lot of time in it. Do this consciously through diet supplementation and technology from now on.

It is a given that as a frequent flyer you are always on the go, therefore the kinds of solutions you need in this and other areas of your lifestyle are solutions that are easier to come by and less energy intensive to apply on your part. With this in mind, the best way to describe the thought that went into choosing protection tools is if you can exercise, eat, drink or sleep you can make these tools work for you. To protect yourself from the flying environment through diet and supplementation make a habit of eating a diet high in quality antioxidants, radio-protective foods, superfoods, enzymes and adaptogens.

As a reminder, let's walk through why it is necessary to see the pesky environment as needing protection against:

- The threat of cosmic radiation equals more exposure to ionizing radiation and an increased risk of cancers.

- The low barometric pressure equals less oxygen in the air, harder for the body to function optimally.

- The dry aircraft cabin equals more dehydration equals more and quicker build-up of acids in the body.

- The low oxygen content equals a more viable environment for germs, pathogens and viruses.

When talking about protection I like to use astronauts as an example. An astronaut would never dream of doing a spacewalk without the protection of his space gear, he knows he wouldn't stand a chance against the elements. When you fly you definitely aren't in space but the environment is equally taxing on the health of your body. You need routine protection, and the last time I checked, wearing a space suit was out of the question! Oh well, I guess we have to settle for the next best thing.

Before we get to the detail in the steps I just want to add that sometimes when you pick up a good how-to book, as you get to the detail that delivers the solution, you may sometimes get apprehensive and ask is this going to work for me? (especially if it's a challenge you've been struggling with for a long time). You might wonder am I going to get it? I know I have! Please don't be overwhelmed by any of the unfamiliar names, terms or nutritional advice given. A quick look in a search engine should help and I will keep the explanation as simple as possible so it is not overwhelming. In the worst case scenario, contact me via the social media channels on the back cover of this book and I'll do my best to help or point you in the right direction.

Step 1: Eat from a wide variety of quality antioxidants, radio-protective foods and enzymes regularly

A high antioxidant diet gives protection from free radicals generated from flying and being in an environment with less than ideal oxygen levels due to barometric pressure. Quenching free radicals with adequate antioxidants will ensure you protect your body and its organs. Choosing the best antioxidants for flyers requires you pick some old favorites and some not so well known ones too. Quality vitamin C is best sourced from non-synthetic origins. These include camu camu (a red/purple cherry-like fruit), which has one of the highest sources of natural vitamin C of any food.

Another good source is the Indian gooseberry (known as Amla) recently dethroned from the number one spot by camu camu. It is important to mention the ongoing discussion about synthetic versus natural vitamin C. Vitamin C in synthetically produced vitamin C products is not the same as naturally food state sourced vitamin C. A look at both types of ascorbic acid (common name for vitamin C) under a microscope lays any doubt to rest. The co-factors that come with natural vitamin C in situ are plain to see while the synthetic variety looks bare in comparison.

Getting the highest quality vitamin C and all its co-factors is what is important so always choose natural sources where possible. Acerola cherries are also noted for a high vitamin C content and are probably easier to come by than camu camu and Indian gooseberry powder. Whatever the case, it is always good to have a constant supply of antioxidants on hand ready to mop up excess free radicals.

High blood serum levels of vitamin C over and above RDA levels have been found to benefit immunity. It is noted that apes in the jungle with naturally high vitamin C levels are immune to viruses and bacteria they easily pick up from contact with the jungle floor. In other words, vitamin C helps them build a robust immune response in the face of compromise; we can benefit from this too by topping up our vitamin C levels.

Side note: Vitamin C is a water-soluble antioxidant. You may also want to consider fat-soluble antioxidants like vitamins A and E as well as carotenoids and lipoic acid.

Other antioxidants worth mentioning are pycnogenol from pine bark extract and glutathione. Pycnogenol is easy to supplement while glutathione is not. Glutathione is tightly regulated so ingestion of glutathione supplements does not raise blood levels. Instead, it is better to eat foods rich in the amino acid cysteine or supplement with N-acetyl cysteine (NAC), curcumin and milk thistle; all of these feed into the glutathione pathway and are better at raising or replenishing it.

Glutathione levels themselves are important to us because of the relationship it has to melatonin. It is thought that glutathione status is indicative of melatonin status. Melatonin levels are important for a good night's sleep, so making sure this super antioxidant is adequately supplied is a priority. Making sure you have enough glutathione for its own sake is also a good move as its role extends much further beyond what is mentioned here.

Radio-protective foods protect the body from the harmful effects of ionizing radiation. They can do this either through their affinity to certain organs in our body or their ability to mop up and bind with some of the free radicals created. For example, iodine naturally found in seaweed is known to protect the thyroid gland. Sodium alginate also in seaweed is known to chelate (bind) radiation free radicals and escort them out of the body. Other radio-protective foods and substances are bee pollen, beets, garlic and clays.

Enzymes are a class of supplements you may be familiar with. Indeed, digestive enzymes are handy for any flyer whose stomach plays up when traveling. More valuable than digestive enzymes are systemic enzymes. The unique quality of enzymes is that they are able to cause biochemical reactions in the body without getting changed themselves. They are like a source of never-ending energy. Because they can do this they are said to have an anti-ageing benefit. Frequent flying is stressful, which accelerates ageing, so using systemic enzymes can have a double benefit. If you are not familiar with them work with a nutritional therapist to guide you on how to get the best out of them.

The bottom line here is to use general and specific supplements and tools to get the results you want. Vitamin C, cysteine-rich foods, beets and clays would count as general supplements while NAC and Pycnogenol and enzymes are examples of more specific ones. The idea of using general and specific tools carries over to another group of nutrients every flyer should have in their arsenal called adaptogens.

Step 2: Invest in a selection of adaptogens

Adaptogens embody this idea of the general and specific perfectly. As well as working through the hypothalamic pituitary adrenal (HPA) axis they have three distinct qualities. Adaptogens are substances that are:

- Non-toxic to the body so they can be taken continually with increasing benefit.

- Non-specific in their mode of action so they always bring the body back to balance but they are specific inasmuch as they are continually reading the body's status.

- Normalizing to the body's systems. Drugs and tonics tend to push the function of the body in one direction or mode of activity; adaptogens always move the body back to balance.

There is a wide range of adaptogens to choose from depending on which part of the world you live in. Some have a more detailed tested and traceable history than others. It is a good idea to stick with these until further validation is available about the newer kids on the block. It is relatively easy to do this without a lot of hands-on knowledge and with a reasonable amount of awareness and caution. The natural healing traditions of Asia, China and India are good starting points. Adaptogens within these traditions have stood the test of time over thousands of years and many have been investigated by scientific methods and been found to be effective.

Adaptogens of specific benefit to flyers due to the exhausting nature of frequent flying include:

- Asian ginseng (root) for adrenal gland exhaustion; the adrenal glands mediate the stress response and are first in the firing line of stress. Often adrenal fatigue results from exhaustion from frequent flying when the flyer is not looking after themselves.

- Holy basil (leaf), Rhodiola (root) and Amla (fruit) benefit the flyer specifically as they are a class of adaptogens that are radio protective. They protect the body from the ever present effects of harmful radiation.

- Astragalus (root) and Licorice (root) help boost immune function through immune modulation and immune stimulation.

- Jiaogulan (leaf) has significant antioxidant activity, which makes it a good inclusion to combat free radical damage, which is accelerated at altitude in oxygen-deficient environments. It has been found to have many of the active ingredients of Asian ginseng.

- Cordyceps (fungi) on account of being able to boost aerobic capacity. The effectiveness of Cordyceps came to light in a big way in 1993 with the performance of some Chinese athletes at the Chinese National Athletics Championships. Athletes were able to set multiple world records due to the benefits of this adaptogen and its ability to increase oxygen efficiency. Drug testing after the event showed no use of banned substances. On a plane in an oxygen-deficient environment Cordyceps is invaluable to those who want to fly well and perform well on arrival.

All of these eight adaptogens are available as tea or powders you can add to meals or snacks. This makes them easy to take with you and consume as needed. The teas even lend themselves to being the perfect accompaniment on the plane. Next time instead of chugging down caffeine and crashing your adrenal glands ask for some hot water and throw a couple of Jiaogulan tea bags in for energy that won't cause you to crash and is kinder on your body (now and long term).

Step 3: Include superfoods in your diet daily

Superfoods – include them using diet and supplementation to protect yourself while in the flying environment and beyond. Certain supermarket chains and supplement companies are fond of labeling entire aisles and the next new thing as superfoods; it can be hard to tell the truth from the hype. One way I've heard superfoods explained is that they are halfway between a medicinal herb and a food. What is certain is that as well as supplying nutrients like regular food they have some extra distinctive strings to their bow. With this in mind let's look at one such distinctive feature of some superfoods that benefit flyers.

The Immunity Feature

Superfoods can build and protect immunity. The easiest way to think of your immune system for the purpose of this explanation is like a lock and key. The immune system has what can be described as docks, which are the locks. Digested nutrients in the foods you eat fit in these docks perfectly as the keys. When a perfect lock and key come together it equals maximum security!

Defining the aircraft cabin as an alien environment makes it a requirement that any of the superfoods we care to consider should have these keys, as our immunity is our first line of defense. Growing and fortifying immunity should be an ongoing priority for every frequent flyer. The great thing about superfoods is they are not limited to just boosting immune function. They are dense sources of nutrients by themselves. They often have distinct antioxidant properties and/or have key nutrients found lacking or in short supply in the general population's diet.

An easy way to start if you are new to superfoods is to pick a few and see how you get on. There are many to choose from but let's look at a few that relate specifically to immunity:

- Goji berries (fruit)
- Spirulina (algae)
- Aloe vera (succulent leaf-like plant)

Glyconutrition is what ties all of these together. Glyco means relating to or producing sugar, so we are talking about sugar nutrition. Before we go any further we must have the understanding that not all sugar is bad for the body. These are types of sugars known as essential sugars. Glyconutrients are long-chain sugars with specific immune-enhancing capability.

Consuming glyconutrients on a regular basis builds and repairs our immunity. Goji berries contain Lycium barbarum polysaccharides (long-chain sugars) touted to be good for immunity and eye health among other things. Spirulina contains a particular polysaccharide complex known as calcium spirulan which is made up of several simple glycosugars all benefiting healthy immune function, and aloe vera contains mannose (a glyconutrient) which is effective at killing yeast.

This is just a fraction of the benefits of some of these superfoods. The uniqueness of superfoods is that they cover so many bases in terms of our requirements. As a busy flyer always on the go, what better way to make sure you are getting quality and quantity nutrition. One of the other great things about superfoods is they are more readily available now than at any other time in our history. As they are more accessible they should become a regular feature in your packing itinerary as you take to the road. For those who are not new to using superfoods it is worthwhile noting that medicinal mushrooms are also very high in glyconutrients so adding them into your diet on a regular basis will also add to the immune fortress you build for yourself as you go about your business. You may want to consider using Reishi, Chaga and Agaricus blazei among others.

SUPERFOOD	USE	SUPERFOOD	USE
Spirulina	Mineral rich	Goji Berries	Essential Sugars
AFA Blue Green Algae	Mineral rich	Cacao	Magnesium ++
Marine Phytoplankton	Mineral rich	Maca	Anti Fatigue +
Aloe Vera	Hydration	Hempseed	Protein + EFA
Coconuts	Hydration	Bee Products	Protein + Enzymes

Inspired by *Superfoods:* David Wolfe

Diagram 3: Top 10 superfoods for flyers

Step 4: Adjust your diet to eating on the alkaline side of the pH scale predominantly

An added form of immunity that often goes unnoticed is blood and body alkalinity status. Naturopathic nutritional therapy teaches that optimum cellular function is achieved when a homeostatic environment is maintained. This relates to the pH level of the blood being maintained within a normal range. For the most part, this tends to be slightly in favor of the alkaline side of the pH scale. In the tissue of the body and the blood when this balance is not maintained trouble starts. The first thing to happen is a derangement of the cellular and surrounding environment, which if not buffered can lead to excess acidity. Acidity, or rather over acidity, is the problem when it occurs in the wrong place.

Over acidity causes cells and blood to function less optimally. This could mean less efficient management of accumulated toxins, which would usually be cleared without any extra resources needed. In the blood specifically a condition known as the Rouleau Effect can occur. This is when the red blood cells clump together because they have lost the charge that normally keeps them apart. As a result, the blood becomes sluggish and doesn't function properly.

If you think about the role of blood as transporting nutrients and moving toxins and other items from one part of the body to another, you begin to see how acidity compromises its function. It is actually the only tissue that has access to all parts, organs and systems of the body. Keeping it clean and functional is really important so it can fulfill its role in the body. With this in mind choosing good blood tonics that clean the blood and revive it are important.

See the Environment step in this section of the book under Alkalize to Energize for suggestions for blood tonics.

The Specific Threat

Ionizing radiation is the elephant in the room flyers are happy to ignore but it deserves a mention with regard to how to protect yourself against its ill effects. Ionizing radiation (IR) has to be considered a threat whether you agree or disagree with its effects, for your health's sake. Why? Because technology makes a difference to how we live now. The always on and connected lifestyle we enjoy means the spread of man-made radiation in all areas of life. The use of Wi-Fi and other radiation sources stress and tax our immunity. Non-ionizing radiation does this to such an extent that we have fewer resources to fight direct cosmic ionizing radiation to which we are exposed when we fly.

Lifestyle goes hand in hand with technology. It is a problem of epidemic proportions. Estimates suggest around 80% of all illnesses relate to the immune function in one way or another. Once upon a time, immune-related disease only accounted for 20% of illnesses. My suspicion is that as we have become a more tech-savvy society, a greater exposure to both types of radiation and less of a connection with our natural habitat is responsible for the decline in immunity. This is another trend set to run for a while yet.

The second wave of Wi-Fi with stronger signals on planes is about to take off. Wi-Fi connectivity in homes is gaining ground too. As technology embeds itself into our lives even more it is potentially increasing our exposure to non-ionizing and ionizing radiation, pushing up the cumulative effect. As the cloud of electropollution continues to engulf the world, everything you can do to protect yourself matters, right down to reducing your exposure to all kinds of radiation and especially so if you fly often. Let us not forget there is no such thing as a safe dose of radiation, no matter what vested interests may want you to believe.

With the trend of increasing modernity and a move away from the rural agricultural age, through the industrial age to the technological age, one thing has remained constant. We have a looser connection to nature and our natural habitat. At a glance this may seem trivial but at its root it holds a truth that is part and parcel of life on this planet.

Just as the rays of the sun nourish us directly and indirectly we are also nourished by the energy fields emanating from the Earth. We are being cut off from these beneficial energies. Modern life, wearing rubber-soled shoes and technology stamp out the connection but getting on a plane literally takes it to another level. It severs it drastically. This is one of the reasons jet lag takes time to adjust to; your body is re-establishing its communication with the Earth, the mother ship.

Step 5: Advanced – invest in grounding technology

As well as moving away from an overly tech lifestyle it is important to create space and balance by regularly establishing your connection with nature. I know it sounds fluffy but being out in nature really does recharge you. If you do this as a habit the worst these harmful electromagnetic fields have to offer will pass you by because you will have tapped into one of the largest sources of inexhaustible antioxidants known to man: negatively charged electrons. These antioxidants neutralize the effects of charged metabolites and tackle inflammation wherever it may be found in the body.

The Earthing Institute is a good source of information for independent research on how tapping into nature is good for your health. They have a range of products that can be adapted to the use of flyers for grounding and help them deal with some aspects of jet lag. Personally I use the recovery bag, which is a sheet-like sleeping bag. All I have to do is plug it into the earth of a socket and I get the benefits of the electrons. Other products they have include:

- Earthing bed sheets

- Earthing pillowcases

- Earthing throws

- Earthing flipflops

- Earthing computer pads and mats

This conversation on technology to help you fly better would not be complete without mentioning the explosion of wearable technology and the tools they put at the disposal of every health-conscious flyer. I have hinted at the good wearables can do for travelers on the go and the capabilities of these gadgets keep expanding. Investing in this type of feedback health tool can serve as a personal coach. Please see this article I wrote about wearable tech a while back, which gives you an idea of what it could do for your travel wellness: Wearable Technology and the Business Traveler:

http://ezinearticles.com/?Wearable-Technology-And-the-Business-Traveller&id=8520548

To some I may have sounded so anti-technology that you won't understand how I can recommend using gadgets like this. To them I say I'm a realist. Whatever tools enable me to find a positive benefit are tools I would consider. My stance is that we need to use technology with caution. Through the P.H.A.R.E. Well program I take active steps to zero out the side effects this and other tech in my life generates, and I urge you to do the same too.

Exercise

After a long-haul flight note how you feel on a scale of 1 to 10, then immediately go find a patch of grass or a body of natural water (whichever is nearest) and stand in it or on it barefoot for 30-45 minutes. When the time is up, use the same 1 to 10 scale and compare. Are you feeling better or worse?

RECAP

Step 1: Eat from a wide variety of quality antioxidants, radio-protective foods and enzymes regularly

Step 2: Invest in a selection of adaptogens

Step 3: Include superfoods in your diet daily

Step 4: Adjust your diet to eating on the alkaline side of the pH scale predominantly

Step 5: Advanced – invest in grounding technology

HYDRATION

Keep Yourself Hydrated

While protecting yourself from the flying environment includes hydration it deserves a category all of its own because hydration does a lot more than just keep our insides wet. The proper functioning of the body is dependent on water as is the conduction of electricity, which is the lifeblood of our ability to function in our bodies. To talk about hydration we have to talk about dehydration because the cabin environment is pressurized and there is less moisture in the cabin air.

You may or may not know that aircraft cabins are pressurized to the kind of air pressure you would expect to find at base camp on your way to the peak of Mount Everest circa 6,000-8,000 feet. This is done gradually during the climb, so while you level out at 36,000 feet the cabin altitude is 6,000-8,000 feet otherwise you would not be able to maintain a comfortable breathing pattern, as the oxygen at that height is thin in the atmosphere.

Planes have air conditioning packs, which help regulate the air drawn off the engines and make it more breathable once it enters the cabin. This helps but it is not ideal; if you've seen a cling film wrapped sandwich exposed on a flight you will notice how quickly the bread becomes stale and hard. The moisture is being sucked out of it just as it is in us! While the new aircraft from Airbus and Boeing have made some strides in comfort, this is still one area yet to be conclusively solved. Indeed, air quality is an issue that underlines the aero-toxic scandal happening at the moment. Every frequent flyer who wants better health while flying would do well to pay attention to the discussion for the sake of their future health.

Performing in Extreme Environments is the title of a book written by Lawrence E. Armstrong (PhD) which looks in detail at the various types of environments athletic activities take place in. Dr. Armstrong goes on to name the different types of groups who may take advantage of the knowledge provided in the book. To his list I would add frequent flyers, especially frequent flyers from the aviation industry who have the cabin environment as their "office." Chapter 5 of the book is worth a read to understand the scope of how altitude affects all of the body's various systems. In the final analysis it leads the reader to the conclusion that action must be taken to overcome the negative effects of altitude on the body for it to work optimally.

Step 1: Stay hydrated throughout your flight

Without being patronizing I would like to point out some properties of water that seem to be lost on most flyers. Its use as a conductor of electricity is what I'm pointing out above but there are others that should occupy our attention. The obvious is water's ability to hydrate. The degree to which hydration happens is partly based on surface tension. All water is not equal in this respect. Surface tension is one of the differences that determine if the water is totally or partially absorbed into the cellular structure it comes into contact with. Put simply, you could drink water with a high surface tension and not be as hydrated as you could be if the surface tension was lower. Surface tension differs between different types of water and other types of fluids you could choose to drink. The lesson is to choose your drinks wisely especially if you are drinking for rehydration purposes.

The effect of altitude on physiology requires flyers take more care about remaining in a positively hydrated state. This is easy to see in less stressful environments than the flying altitude. Over the past few years you may have seen or read the horror stories of athletes fainting on the field of play due to dehydration. As I write there is discussion at FIFA whether to move the 2022 Qatar World Cup games to winter for fear of the brutal dehydrating summer weather in Qatar. The message is simple: dehydration impairs performance. Dehydration leads to sluggish elimination, which encourages toxins to accumulate and further jams up the gears of the body. If not corrected it encourages ill health to settle in.

This step of the program is so important because it is so simple and yet so widely ignored by most flyers. People are too quick to point to horror stories like the one where actor Anthony Andrews drank too much water and diluted the sodium in his body (hyponatremia). They point to this kind of anomaly without acknowledging that flying constantly dehydrates you. In any event, making sure you have adequate sodium from the diet you eat regularly would guard against hyponatremia.

The dehydration effect on flyers is not helped by the hydration choices provided by the airlines, or liquid restrictions imposed by civil aviation authorities in a post 9/11 flying environment. In some instances airlines are themselves the perpetrators as they offer you wine, liquor and caffeinated beverages and recommend they be consumed in moderation! On an aircraft with its harsh drying environment, asking for moderation is misplaced. Flyers need to be educated about the real effects of these drinks at altitude and discouraged from taking them for the sake of their well-being.

The general perception of flying is that it is glamorous and elite. The flying experience is seen to start immediately on boarding (or in the business lounge) and as soon as the first bottle of champagne or wine is offered. Most flyers expect to be indulged in some way or another and airlines are not blind to this so they encourage it. Now that the flying habit has been around for 90 plus years and we know how it affects health, this romantic view of flying must be replaced with the realization that the flying experience is not the aim of taking the journey. Getting drunk just before or during a flight for whatever reason is no longer an option. This is especially so for frequent flyers on business or any other kind of frequent flyer.

Step 2: Get structured water tools

The view that science is coming around to is that the water held in biological systems (like our physiology) is structured. That is to say it is ordered in such a way that it helps the cells work properly; some would say that it is ordered to reduce impedance and allow the best flow of electrical current between cells thereby encouraging maximum functionality.

Early research in this field done by Dr. Gerald Pollack, a professor of bioengineering at the University of Washington, is promising. His book *Cells, Gels and the Engines of Life* goes into detail about his findings in which water plays a central role when it is structured. On the other side of the debate is the argument that water-cleaning plants for all their good intentions remove this structure from the water during processing. As a result, the water most of us use has lost its structure and requires effort to be restructured if it is to be of maximum benefit. When this happens it is less than optimal.

How do you get more structured water into your body for the purpose of better health while flying? Well, without going into a long-winded explanation of all the properties of structured water, an easy way to get a handle on it is to do one or a few of the following things:

- Install a water purifying system in your home, which structures all the water you use.

- Juice as a lifestyle choice. Water from organic fresh fruits and vegetables ticks all the boxes of what makes structured water.

- Supplement with hydrogen – see Dr. Flanagan mentioned below.

Dr. Pollack refers to some natural sources of structured water in an online interview with Dr. Joseph Mercola, for example the waters at Lourdes in France and some of the waters of the Ganges in the Himalayas. Dr. Patrick Flanagan is another scientist who has researched the properties of water (of the Hunza region of Pakistan) and produced a product that mimics these natural sources of structured water. As a standby or last resort it is good to have this supplement to hand when traveling to help you stay hydrated. Go to www.phisciences.com for details of Megahydrate.

Personally I think a combination of all three examples is best. The sidebar to this is that as you start to increase the amount of structured water in your diet, you will start to eliminate more toxins from your body so caution should be observed. Go at a manageable pace to avoid excessive unmanageable detoxification symptoms. If you do find yourself with unmanageable symptoms like headaches and nausea, find a detoxification practitioner to work with to ease the transition.

For hydration purposes I have used the following tools with success and recommend you try them:

- Aquathin home water purification system

- Megahydrate supplement

- Crystal Energy supplement

- Hydrogen Boost supplement

- Water-to-Go water bottle with a NASA space program designed filter

A common theme in the topic of hydration is the role of hydrogen. In fact all we are trying to do is introduce more negatively charged hydrogen into the body. Whether you do it with water which has two molecules of hydrogen to one of oxygen (H_2O) or with a predominantly carbohydrate meal where carbohydrates are made up of multiple chains of carbon, hydrogen and oxygen (CHO), the important thing is to get hydrated and stay that way throughout your flight. As a bare minimum, if you can't, won't or don't use any of the other tools, eating a high-carb meal before your flight or during your flight may be of some benefit.

Exercise

Test this for yourself. On your next couple of flights take a pack of pH testing strips with you, you can order them online or buy them in any decent health food store. Test your urine pH by dipping the paper in the flow as you urinate:

(a) before you get on the flight

(b) after the meal service

(c) after you have slept inflight

(d) when you get off the flight

You will see how dehydrating and disruptive the flying environment is. You will also find that if you are particularly active during the flight your urine will turn yellow more quickly (indicating acidity). Of course, if you are on any medications with dye in them or B vitamin supplements these will mask the evidence of dehydration.

In closing, every time you go to board a plane it should conjure up images of a parched desert with the scorching sun beating down on you, zero humidity and fierce dry winds. Who among us would dare attempt to make a journey in these conditions without being adequately prepared? This is the challenge for every frequent flyer: protect yourself and be prepared for the deceptively harsh environment of the plane whenever you fly.

RECAP

Step 1: Stay hydrated throughout your flight
Step 2: Get structured water tools

ACCLIMATIZATION

Get on Local Time as Soon as Possible

Acclimatization is accomplished in superficial and simple ways. In the airline industry, for flight attendants and pilots specifically, the amount of time spent at a destination is deemed as enough time to have acclimatized. This is one of the reasons the time allowed at various destinations around the globe differs.

There are accelerators and decelerators of acclimatization, which flyers can use to their advantage if they so choose. The simplest accelerator is to connect with your new environment and the simplest decelerator is to stay disconnected from the new environment. The surest way to master acclimatizing regardless of how often you fly is to become adept at reconnecting to the natural energies of our ideal environment, the Earth. Meditation, deep breathing, going barefoot and brain entraining tools are also good choices to accomplish this, depending on your situation, time constraints and circumstances.

Step 1: Raise your core temperature and sync with your surroundings with Zeitgebers

In chronobiology (study of rhythms in biological systems) the surest way to know a body has returned to normal after jet lag is through body temperature adjustment. Temperature is the last marker to return to normal. Research also shows that willfully resetting your body clock is possible by using exercise (among other things) that causes your core temperature to rise, thus forcing a reset. This is one more reason to hard-wire exercise into your lifestyle.

Another way of looking at the flying experience is to view the flyer's body as having lost its sense of direction after each flight. Being out of touch with the environment is like having no frame of reference as to where you are and not knowing what to do. Think about it like this: if you were dropped off in a jungle or a desert and you touched a poisonous plant or were without sun protection you would suffer the consequences. You wouldn't blend in; you wouldn't know what to do and what not to do to get in sync. Landing anywhere and not being able to blend into the time zone environment means you are going to get punished too.

The punishment comes in the many symptoms that make up jet lag and being out of sync. On the other hand, if you knew how to distinguish desert flora and fauna and you knew the desert dwellers' methods of finding water and seeking shade you would be able to thrive in these conditions. Mastering acclimatization is similar: if you know what distinctions to look out for, encourage or discourage, you can arrive and blend in without much effort.

The science of chronobiology goes some way to help us identify groups of these distinctions to help us master our environments. Some of the most important ones are called Zeitgebers or time givers. They are cues and clues we take from our environment which inform us on multiple levels what time it is in relationship to our environment. The strongest Zeitgeber is the alternate lightness and darkness in the 24-hour cycle; others include mealtimes, and there is another class known as social Zeitgebers, which include the normal times you might spend interacting and carrying out the functions of a normal day. The best way to put these to use when you arrive at your destination is to get into the general flow of what the locals are doing, so if it is lunchtime go to lunch, if it is bedtime go to bed. It is, as the saying goes, when in Rome do as the Romans do.

RECAP

Step 1: Raise your core temperature and sync with your surroundings with Zeitgebers

RHYTHMS

Run Your Body Clock Naturally

The world we live in is full of rhythm. While it is easy to see this rhythm in nature it is also part and parcel of us. The story of Heracles is an analogy worth noting in this respect. In Greek mythology Heracles defeats Antaeus (half giant) on his way to the garden of Hesperides to perform his 11th labor. Heracles is only able to defeat Antaeus, son of Poseidon and Gaia, by holding him aloft from the earth in a bear hug.

Antaeus's power came from the connection he had with his mother (Gaia) the Earth, and so it is with the human race in more ways than one. Essentially our well-being is dependent on our connection with the Earth. When you fly you sever this connection and it needs to be reconnected. This is the essence of Rhythms, getting back into harmony with our natural environment.

Even though the geomagnetic properties of the Earth's atmosphere are unseen they play an important role in our health. Some if not most of the biological functions we take for granted are encouraged by our connection with the rhythm of our environment. Hormonal action is an example of this. Hormones help us maintain the rhythm of life in our bodies through their regulatory actions.

The most talked-about hormone in relation to healthy flying and jet lag is of course melatonin. It is important to note a couple of things about melatonin. The first is that as well as its regulatory function it is a super antioxidant. It has cachet value in this respect all on its own especially for frequent flyers. Secondly, like all hormones it works in the body in concert with other hormones, or to put it more precisely, all hormones work within a biofeedback mechanism, which means the presence of one affects the presence and function of others. This is important to know because the standard answer to the problems of jet lag is to supplement with melatonin without regard to the potential upset this will cause to other hormones in the body.

Step 1: Supplement specifically to prime the melatonin pathway

Melatonin's role in controlling the body clock is well established so it deserves our attention; however, focusing on melatonin alone or the body clock alone is not a viable long-term solution. If you supplement it directly you run the risk of upsetting your hormonal balance in other respects over time.

The path to melatonin production looks like this:

Tryptophan —— 5HTP —— Serotonin —— Melatonin

As a nutritional therapist my chosen approach would be to use supplements and foods that prime the melatonin pathway while making sure you get out and expose yourself to sunlight on a consistent basis as a lifestyle habit. Do this by eating foods high in tryptophan and melatonin (see tables below).

Tryptophan

- Game meat - Spirulina

- Spinach - Soy Protein Isolate

- Sesame seeds - Egg whites - Turkey

- Watercress - Halibut - Crab

Natural Melatonin (preferable to synthetic)

- Tart cherries - Walnuts

- Mustard seeds - Corn

- Rice - Ginger root

Tart cherries stand head and shoulders above any of the other foods for melatonin and should be a regular addition to your diet. After that walnuts are a distant second. Walnuts contain omega 3 essential fatty acids which help in reducing inflammation so are a worthwhile addition for that reason alone.

Step 2: Practice the same sleep routine

For the sake of simplicity, the media painted cortisol as the stress hormone and a bad guy, but that is not the sum total of the function of cortisol in the body. Did you know that healthy cortisol secretions have an inverse relationship with melatonin? When melatonin rises in the evening to prepare you for sleep, cortisol declines only to rise to its peak around the time you get up. It helps you wake up. So you can see that if you are stressed before you go to bed, sleep onset primed by melatonin is less likely to take place in a hurry.

To play it safe and in keeping with the title of this section (Rhythms) it makes sense to develop good sleep rhythms/ protocols to ensure restful sleep. This means no late-night pulse-raising movies, no harsh lighting including computer and smartphone screens and no heavy disagreeable meals. A quiet, clean, uncluttered sleeping space with no noise distractions is what is required. The important thing is to go to sleep the same way every night. Do the same helpful things so your body recognizes the cues you send it and knows what to do. Even if travel doesn't allow for sleeping the same time every night, decent sleep routines should be practiced to send your body the message that you are prepping for sleep.

Step 3: Mega dose vitamin C

In its role as a stress hormone, when blood levels of cortisol rise in response to stress vitamin C levels decline. Supplementing and eating a diet high in vitamin C will help keep stress-induced cortisol levels in check and thus in rhythm. This is practical advice for anyone who doesn't sleep well on the plane or any flyer who finds the whole flying process exhausting. Make vitamin C supplementation a daily part of your wellness program over and above RDAs. Vitamin C is water soluble so any overdose you have will pass out of the body through urine.

Step 4: Use technology to get in sync

In addition to supplements and diet, technology offers some useful tools every frequent flyer should make use of in order to maintain the healthy rhythm of living that flying disrupts. The most hated kind of disruption frequent flyers dread is disruption to sleep. Once you've sorted your diet and sleep routine in steps 1 and 2 above, turn to brainwave technology for extra help. This is a quick primer:

- Beta wave - 12.5 to 30 Hz – normal waking consciousness

- Alpha wave - 8 to 15 Hz – relaxed meditative alertness

- Theta wave - 4 to 7 Hz – level at which healing is purported to take place

- Delta wave - 0.1 to 3 Hz – deep dreamless sleep, level at which if woken grogginess is experienced

For our purposes the most interesting brainwaves are the alpha and theta ranges as they facilitate relaxation, rest and healing. Being able to induce or entrain the mind to produce these brainwaves is handy for being more productive and adapting a broken sleep schedule.

Getting back into the rhythm is as simple as going to the mountaintop for 10 years and mastering the art of quieting the mind! If you don't happen to have a handy mountaintop nearby, brainwave apps are handy alternatives. Coupled with a pair of noise-canceling headphones they make it easy for anyone with 15 minutes or more to get back in tune (entrain). Note: this is also some of the good technology can do for frequent flyers I've mentioned earlier in the book!

Step 5: Advanced – meridian tracing

As well as having external prompts to keep us in rhythm we have internalized rhythm too. In Chinese traditional medicine evidence of this is to be found in the meridian wheel, the natural cycle of influence the twelve meridians have in the body. (Meridians are energy pathways of the body). The cycle mirrors the functioning of a clock in that the energy in a meridian comes into prominence one after another for a two-hour period and then moves on to the next meridian.

It is my hypothesis that if the body did not know what time it was due to having spent so much time flying, influencing the body by connecting with the energy of the meridians is a way to get the body back into rhythm and cut jet lag short. Tracing the central and governing meridians serves to reset the body followed by tracing the meridian of the hour. See the work of Donna Eden in recommended reading for further details.

In summary, the rhythm step is all about having an understanding of jet lag which acknowledges that flying constantly upsets your natural rhythms and having the tools to reset these rhythms on an ongoing basis. Making these resetting habits part of your daily life is the easiest way to do this. Diet, supplements and brainwave apps are some of the tools at your disposal.

RECAP

Step 1: Supplement specifically to prime the melatonin pathway

Step 2: Practice the same sleep routine

Step 3: Mega dose vitamin C

Step 4: Use technology to get in sync

Step 5: Advanced 1 – meridian tracing

ENVIRONMENTS

Master Your Environment

It is true to say that mankind's success at living in the variable climates that exist on Earth boils down to some degree of mastery of the environment. When we are encapsulated in a metal tube flying at 36,000 feet above the Earth the same rules apply but this tends to be forgotten. Preparing for flying with this knowledge in mind is the difference between those who fly well by design and those who get by perchance.

Step 1: Master your inner terrain

The cabin environment is not what we think it to be. In fact we take it for granted in many of the habits and things we do when we fly. It wasn't too long ago that it was okay to smoke on a plane in an environment that had less oxygen than we have at sea level. Airlines make a point of signing famous chefs to make signature dishes the palate cannot fully appreciate at altitude because of a 25% loss of taste in the sky. Serving alcohol is another practice flyers are accustomed to which contradicts any notion of healthy flying.

If that were not enough, airlines are busying themselves fitting in-flight Wi-Fi on planes without the consideration that an enclosed space in the sky is not the place to encourage the use of devices that use non-ionizing radiation and give off emissions. In the face of the effects these conditions create, your inner terrain is your only defense. You must learn to fortify and manage it as a way of life for you to stand a better chance of flying well.

From my perspective, diet is the best way to manage your inner terrain; however, it is important to know that thoughts and mental states of mind also create stress, which has negative impacts on it. Therefore paying attention to our thought patterns and feelings is invaluable too.

Alkalize to Energize

Broadly speaking, looking after your inner terrain is about the ability to stay alkaline enough to function and have extra capacity to buffer excess acidity that comes your way. Green plant matter has the ability to do this better than all other classes of food due to its chlorophyll content and the fact that it is mineral rich. Under the microscope chlorophyll is almost identical to blood save for the central molecule. Chlorophyll has magnesium at its center and hemoglobin has iron at the center of its molecule.

Blood pH is the marker we want to keep an eye on. Factors that affect the pH of our blood range from respiration to diet to activity or a lack of activity and more. They relate to the blood's function as moving tissue and the fact that it has a detoxifying role. It can take toxins created in the body and move them to sites where they can be voided and expelled. Flying in an environment with a lack of oxygen, poor air quality and acidifying food and beverage choices burdens the body and interferes with the detoxifying role the blood has to other organs and parts of the body.

Chlorophyll cleanses the blood making it more alkaline, so mother was right, you should eat your greens, as a frequent flyer you should juice them too. If you didn't have a reason to eat your greens before, you do now. If you are going to make it a regular thing it bears repeating that it is an uphill battle as it takes about 20 parts alkalinity to buffer one part acidity. Some great alkalizing plants for juicing and food are:

- Wheatgrass - Barley grass - Swiss chard - Kelp

- Spinach - Kale - Watercress - Mint - Parsley

- Mustard greens - Lettuce - Dandelion greens

- Wakame seaweed - Collards - Green cabbage

- Sunflower greens

Supplement your diet to cover your extra nutrient requirements

Frequent flying does something else to the flyer: it drains them of nutrients. The lack of nutrients may come about through the body protecting itself when you fly or through neglect in the kinds of meals you feed yourself as a result of the lifestyle. Whatever the case, the cellular environment needs more nutrients just to keep functioning properly. By necessity this environment should be fed a diet rich in minerals and trace nutrients on a regular basis.

Maintaining a healthy cellular environment by supplying these nutrients in abundance works in another important way. When these nutrients are missing not only does it play havoc with the proper functioning of the organ or system of the body but it also opens the door for possible radioactive analogue isotopes (similar to the required nutrient but radioactive) to fill the deficiency. For example, if you don't have enough iodine in your diet it is possible that your body might choose to store iodine 131, a radioactive form of iodine, in its place because that is what's on hand. If or when this occurs it can disrupt organ functions and spread oxidation within the organ or system. Making sure these nutrient requirements were met in the first place could have prevented this altogether.

There is a parallel story for antioxidants: large amounts of antioxidants are required to mop up any absorbed radiation free radicals created. A low antioxidant intake potentially exposes you to more cellular damage. Since some radiation isotopes can have a long lifespan it is advisable to keep antioxidant levels high as a lifestyle choice or at least for as long as you are a frequent flyer. It is handy to remember that these are requirements over and above what your body needs for its normal functioning. It would be wise to look beyond RDAs depending on your constitution and level of activity.

RECAP

Step 1: Master your biochemistry

- Alkalize to energize

- Supplement your diet to cover your extra
  nutrient requirements

WELLNESS

Build Vitality on the Road

We all know that frequent flying is physically demanding. The only sure way to overcome this aspect of flying is to become fitter as well as healthier. Fitness will help you deal with the rigors of the journey better and will also enable you to enjoy a better quality of life if you take fitness to heart and make it part of your lifestyle. This is exactly what I am advocating here and there is good reason to recommend this approach.

The first reason has to do with one of the training effects you get from regular exercise if it is done properly. VO2 Max is a measurement of how efficiently your body uses oxygen. When you exercise on a regular basis you can train your body to become more efficient at utilizing oxygen. This comes in very handy when you think about the cabin environment; it is a place with less than optimal oxygen compared to sea level. Being able to utilize what oxygen there is efficiently will give you an advantage over any untrained fellow travelers and allow you to arrive in better shape than them.

The second reason to take exercise to heart is that scientific research is confirming the benefits of aerobic exercise to help reset the body clock. If you Google the article *The biological clock keeps ticking but exercise may turn it back*, it reports on preliminary research done with mice. Aerobic exercise done for a set duration involves raising your core temperature. As mentioned above, the field of chronobiology has discovered that core temperature is the last marker of the body clock to reset and signifies a resynchronization of the body to its environment. Raising the core temperature through aerobic exercise is a shortcut to make that vital reset happen sooner with no downside. If you are a frequent flyer, executing an exercise plan on a regular basis ought to be a lifestyle no-brainer decision.

Step 1: Train for the road

The best way to implement an exercise plan is to start with something easy you like doing especially if you are starting from scratch. It is better to choose something you can sustain rather than jump in the deep end and lose interest down the road. Once the habit is in place you can mix it up and start some other types of exercise for variety and additional benefits. I have found that a mix of aerobic, resistance and soft martial arts exercises cover all the requirements I have while on the road. While we tend to think of exercise as an all-out assault in the gym or workout space, the truth is we need to balance intensity with energy, rest and recuperation. Having a variety of exercises to turn to helps you get this balance and keep it by alternating what you choose to do.

Step 2: Detox on a regular basis

Another aspect of wellness that is important to the healthy frequent flyer is detoxification. A true frequent flyer travels the world and is exposed to many different environments all the time. To be able to deal with whatever the physical environment presents to you requires you to keep your immunity in top form. One of the easiest ways to do this is to create a periodic detoxification regimen for yourself.

Find out what suits you best, what kinds of therapies or treatments you can comfortably do and invest in them. Besides the actual physiological benefit they will bring it will also increase your sense of well-being and reduce stress. The more you do it, the more you teach your body to let go and use eustress to get the upper hand in health. The sense of nurturing is always important for anyone who often travels away from home.

The background to helping wellness show up in your life as a function of healthy flying requires you to see the solution to jet lag and travel weariness as a lifestyle challenge more than anything else. The more you accept this as a fact of your life, the easier it will be to plan ahead in your affairs and have the different areas of your life strategically aligned with flying, without them clashing or detracting from the wellness path you are on.

I can use one example to show you what I mean. Most flyers know it is important to stay hydrated; however, for a lot of people that thought only pops into their head when they are on the plane. While this is better than nothing, the best long-term view would be to really understand the dynamics that make up good quality hydrating water and invest in a home pure water system solution in advance. That way you incorporate it into your lifestyle even when you are not flying. Alternatively, if that were not an option and you understood the principle of structured water you might decide to invest in a juicing regimen and get your structured water from fruits and vegetables on a regular basis.

The most important thing about the wellness aspect of this program is to work with your strengths, strengthen and build upon your weaknesses. We all have health and physiologies that are unique, it is important to bear this in mind when considering a wellness program so you can get the best results for yourself. If you look at travelers and frequent flyers today you will notice that one ingredient is almost universally lacking: vitality is in short supply because most of the tools flyers use to stay on track while on the road drain it. Looking after your wellness on purpose will help you avoid this trap but you have to do it from the ground up, not just as a solution to the temporary itch of jet lag but as a lifestyle that gives you vitality in everything else you do.

In summary, the Wellness step is about the steps you are prepared to take on a regular basis to nurture your health. It includes exercise, the diet you habitually consume to stay healthy, the general and specific supplements you use to buffer the demands of your chosen lifestyle, the use of technology as an enabler of success and the way you prioritize your workload to avoid overwhelm that is so common among frequent flyers.

RECAP

Step 1: Train for the road

Step 2: Detox on a regular basis

Farewell!

So there you have it, we have arrived with the smoothest of touchdowns! You are now set to cruise to your hotel for that meeting, event, vacation or rest. You are safe in the knowledge that no matter what the journey may bring, you can meet it head on without digging into your reserves of energy and burning out. When others are failing you are just getting started. You took the time to rebuild from the ground up. Bravo.

Presence is that feeling jam-packed with health, vitality and a feeling of being in control. The better you fly, the more you will be able to exercise your presence for your benefit and the purpose of your travel. The tools in part two are to help you build that presence in bucketloads. Dive in and unleash your best self yet.

I would like to leave you with one thought: man has made voyages and traveled the Earth from ancient times, be it the Trans Saharan trade routes, the Silk Road trade routes or religious pilgrimages. They did it artfully and over long periods of time. They learned much about the world and themselves in the process. Flying in the 21st century still holds that promise – to learn about the world and ourselves – and it requires us to be at our best.

Health is one of those tools that supports us being our best and these tools are an offering to make it possible. Use them wisely and watch them go to work for you here and in every other area of your life.

Wherever you go, P.H.A.R.E. Well!

References

INTRODUCTION

FDA rejects jet lag drug by Cephalon - NYT.
com http://www.nytimes.com/2010/03/30/
business/30drug.html

Power Pills - Business Traveler magazine Asia
http://www.businesstraveller.asia/asia-pacific/
archive/2011/december-2011/special-reports/
power-pills

CHAPTER 1 - WHAT CAN FREQUENT FLYERS
LEARN FROM SAVVY PILOTS AND CREW?

Burnout –The Latest Fashion - World Economic
Forum –http://www.we**forum**.org/videos/
burnout-latest-fashion

CHAPTER 2 - JET LAG NEEDS A NEW
CONVERSATION

Melatonin - Melatonin.com
http://melatonin.com/melatonin-cautions.php

Flight non-attendants - Journal of Neuroscience
http://www.nature.com/news/2000/000315/full/
news000316-8.html

The California Institute for Human Science – Ghaly M. & Teplitz D.

The biologic effects of grounding the human body during sleep as measured by cortisol levels and subjective reporting of sleep, pain and stress. Journal of Alternative Complementary Medicine 10 (5): 767-776, 2004

CHAPTER 3 - THE DETERMINANTS OF JET LAG

American Express Business Traveler Survey 2007 http://www.newbusiness.co.uk/articles/travel-advice/stresses-business-travel-uncovered

McClintock Effect - http://en.wikipedia.org/wiki/Menstrual_synchrony

CHAPTER 4 - THE P.H.A.R.E. WELL SYSTEM OF JET LAG ELIMINATION AND PREVENTION

US economy loses $70 billion in productivity due to jet lag annually http://www.bloomberg.com/video/57035632-cephalon-s-nuvigil-for-jet-lag-awaits-fda-approval.html

CHAPTER 5 - WHY THE P.H.A.R.E. WELL SYSTEM IS AN IDEA WHOSE TIME HAS COME FOR FREQUENT FLYERS

Argonne Institute Anti Jet Lag Diet http://www.netlib.org/misc/jet-lag-diet

CHAPTER 6 - WHY FLYING HAS CHANGED AND SO MUST YOU

The Future for Interurban Passenger Transport - Bringing Citizens Closer Together. International Transport Research Symposium of 2009

The Bottom Line with Evan Davis – Travel http://www.radiotimes.com/episode/w4ddd/the-bottom-line--episode-3-travel

A Briefing Report on Autoimmune Diseases and AARDA: Past Present and Future - National Autoimmune Diseases Summit: The Global State of Autoimmunity Today

Grants for electrosensitives http://www.mastsanity. org/health-52/sweden-: -ehs-peoples-rights-to-an-accessible-society.html

Mobile Dependence: A Growing Trend in Business Travel http://www.pchousing.com/blog/968/pc-housing-infographic-mobile-dependence-a-growing-trend-in-business-travel

CHAPTER 7 - CHALLENGES UNIQUE TO FREQUENT FLYERS

Adrenal Fatigue https://www.adrenalfatigue.org/what-is-adrenal-fatigue

CHAPTER 8 - THE OUTCOMES OF A JETSPERT

A Jetspert - a made-up word, which distinguishes a frequent flyer who is able to travel the globe, be fully present and not suffer the effects of jet lag when called upon to do business, leisure activities or perform. Trademarked to Nucentricals Ltd.

Recomendations &
Further Reading

Adaptogens: Herbs for Strength, Stamina and Stress Relief – David Winston & Steven Maimes

Adrenal Fatigue, The 21st Century Stress Syndrome – James L. Wilson.

The Ancient Wisdom of the Chinese Tonic Herbs – Ron Teeguarden

Alkalize or Die – Dr. Theodore A. Baroody

The Body Electric – Robert O. Becker & Gary Selden

Earthing, the most important health discovery ever? – Clint Ober, Stephen T. Sinatra M.D. & Martin Zucker

Fighting Radiation and Chemical Pollutants with Food, Herbs and Vitamins – Steven R. Schechter N.D.

Performing in Extreme Environments – Lawrence E. Armstrong PhD

Superfoods – David Wolfe

Weaving The Energies: Setting the field – The Workbook - Donna Colleen Eden

SUMMARY

PROTECTION

Step 1: Eat from a wide variety of antioxidants, radio-protective foods and enzymes regularly

Step 2: Invest in a selection of adaptogens

Step 3: Include superfoods in your diet daily

Step 4: Adjust your diet to eating on the alkaline side of the pH scale predominantly

Step 5: Advanced – invest in grounding technology

HYDRATION

Step 1: Stay hydrated throughout your flight

Step 2: Get structured water tools

ACCLIMATIZATION

Step 1: Raise your core temperature and sync with your surroundings with Zeitgebers

RHYTHMS

Step 1: Supplement specifically to prime the melatonin pathway

Step 2: Practice the same sleep routine

Step 3: Mega dose vitamin C

Step 4: Use technology to get in sync

Step 5: Advanced 1 – meridian tracing

ENVIRONMENTS

Step 1: Master your biochemistry

- Alkalize to energize

- Supplement your diet to cover your extra nutrient requirements

WELLNESS

Step 1: Train for the road

Step 2: Detox on a regular basis

About the Author

Christopher is a flight attendant, nutritional therapist and frequent flyer. Having flown for a combination of 17 years for a major airline on long- and short-haul fleets, he brings knowledge, experience, expertise and insight to the book you now hold in your hands.

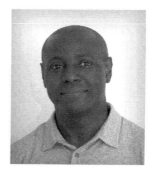

As a nutritional therapist who can count British Airways cabin crew as private clients he has dealt with frequent flying, jet lag and its consequences at their most brutal. As a therapist running a private jet lag clinic Chris has seen first-hand the impact frequent flying has on business travelers' health and productivity. As an entrepreneur himself Chris has experienced the toll of jet lag before creating the P.H.A.R.E. Well System of jet lag elimination and prevention.

As a co-founder of Global Business Travel Wellness Advisors (GBTWA) Chris shares the passion to change the way people fly by educating and informing the traveling public on how to travel well and healthily, long term.

This book shows you, the jet-lagged flyer, how to master all the variables of flying well. It introduces you to tools you can make use of right now as well as tools you can incorporate into your lifestyle. It outlines the six easy steps any flyer can use that go beyond popping pills, caffeine and alcohol to beat jet lag. Chris is a firm believer in useful practical knowledge and brings this approach to the methodology in this book.

Chris's present and past contributions to the ongoing conversation about healthy flying include blogs, articles and video content on YouTube, SlideShare, Facebook and LinkedIn. You can connect with him and his content at @ thejetspert on Twitter, Friends of a Jet Lag Free World on Facebook and as an expert author for EzineArticles.com under the Business Travel section.